Sports Nutrition for Masters Athletes

Sports Nutrition for Masters Athletes

Peter G. Nickless, DC, PhD
Dean of Online Education
Director Master of Science in Applied Clinical Nutrition
Northeast College of Health Sciences
Seneca Falls, NY, USA

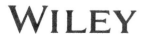

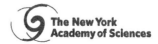

Copyright © 2025 by John Wiley & Sons, Inc. All rights reserved, including rights for text and data mining and training of artificial technologies or similar technologies.

Published by John Wiley & Sons, Inc., Hoboken, New Jersey.
Published simultaneously in Canada.

No part of this publication may be reproduced, stored in a retrieval system, or transmitted in any form or by any means, electronic, mechanical, photocopying, recording, scanning, or otherwise, except as permitted under Section 107 or 108 of the 1976 United States Copyright Act, without either the prior written permission of the Publisher, or authorization through payment of the appropriate per-copy fee to the Copyright Clearance Center, Inc., 222 Rosewood Drive, Danvers, MA 01923, (978) 750-8400, fax (978) 750-4470, or on the web at www.copyright.com. Requests to the Publisher for permission should be addressed to the Permissions Department, John Wiley & Sons, Inc., 111 River Street, Hoboken, NJ 07030, (201) 748-6011, fax (201) 748-6008, or online at http://www.wiley.com/go/permission.

Trademarks: Wiley and the Wiley logo are trademarks or registered trademarks of John Wiley & Sons, Inc. and/or its affiliates in the United States and other countries and may not be used without written permission. All other trademarks are the property of their respective owners. John Wiley & Sons, Inc. is not associated with any product or vendor mentioned in this book.

Limit of Liability/Disclaimer of Warranty: While the publisher and author have used their best efforts in preparing this book, they make no representations or warranties with respect to the accuracy or completeness of the contents of this book and specifically disclaim any implied warranties of merchantability or fitness for a particular purpose. No warranty may be created or extended by sales representatives or written sales materials. The advice and strategies contained herein may not be suitable for your situation. You should consult with a professional where appropriate. Further, readers should be aware that websites listed in this work may have changed or disappeared between when this work was written and when it is read. Neither the publisher nor authors shall be liable for any loss of profit or any other commercial damages, including but not limited to special, incidental, consequential, or other damages.

For general information on our other products and services or for technical support, please contact our Customer Care Department within the United States at (800) 762-2974, outside the United States at (317) 572-3993 or fax (317) 572-4002.

Wiley also publishes its books in a variety of electronic formats. Some content that appears in print may not be available in electronic formats. For more information about Wiley products, visit our web site at www.wiley.com.

Library of Congress Cataloging-in-Publication Data
Names: Nickless, Peter G., author.
Title: Sports nutrition for masters athletes / Peter G. Nickless.
Description: Hoboken, New Jersey : Wiley, [2025] | Includes index.
Identifiers: LCCN 2024028315 (print) | LCCN 2024028316 (ebook) | ISBN 9781119904304 (paperback) | ISBN 9781119904311 (adobe pdf) | ISBN 9781119904328 (epub)
Subjects: LCSH: Athletes–Nutrition.
Classification: LCC TX361.A8 N53 2025 (print) | LCC TX361.A8 (ebook) | DDC 613.202/4796–dc23/eng/20240723
LC record available at https://lccn.loc.gov/2024028315
LC ebook record available at https://lccn.loc.gov/2024028316

Cover Design: Wiley
Cover Images: © PeopleImages.com - Yuri A/Shutterstock, © Westend61/Getty Images, © vm/Getty Images, © Photo and Co/Getty Images

Set in 9.5/12.5pt STIXTwoText by Straive, Pondicherry, India

SKY10082731_082324

I decicate this book to my family: my wife Katie, daughters Samantha, Nicole, and Vivian and my grandchildren Jacob and Charlie. You are the reason why I do everything I do. You are my inspiration and my support. Thank you for putting up with me during the writing of this book.

I would also like to dedicate this book to my brother and to all of the master's athletes. This book is for all of you still woking to be your best and not giving up on your dreams at any age.

Contents

Preface *xv*

1 Overview *1*
1.1 Introduction *1*
1.2 Demographic Data *2*
1.3 What Is Sports Nutrition? *3*
1.4 Why Study Sports Nutrition? *3*
1.5 What Is a Masters Athlete? *4*
1.6 Why Focus on Masters Athletes? *4*
1.7 What Are the Nutrients Used by Athletes? *5*
1.8 Macronutrients *6*
1.9 Micronutrients *6*
1.10 Hydration *7*
1.11 Supplementation *7*
1.12 Overview: A Nutrient Approach to Diet *8*
1.13 Conclusion *10*
References *11*

2 A Biochemistry and Physiology *13*
2.1 Introduction *13*
2.2 Homeostasis *14*
2.3 Energy Production *15*
2.3.1 Forms of Energy *16*
2.4 Biochemical Reactions in Sports Nutrition *16*
2.4.1 Glycolysis *17*
2.4.2 Beta-oxidation *17*
2.4.3 Gluconeogenesis *17*
2.4.4 Tricarboxylic Acid Cycle *18*

2.4.5 Ketogenesis *18*
2.4.6 Glycogenesis *18*
2.4.7 Glycogenolysis *18*
2.5 Energy Systems *19*
2.5.1 What Are Energy Systems? *20*
2.5.2 Phosphagen System *20*
2.5.3 Anaerobic Glycolysis *21*
2.5.4 Aerobic Glycolysis *22*
2.5.5 Intensity *22*
2.5.6 Case Study – Jim *24*
2.6 Conclusion *25*
References *25*

3 The Aging Process *27*
3.1 Introduction *27*
3.2 Performance-Based Changes *28*
3.3 Motor Neuron Changes *29*
3.4 Endocrine Changes *30*
3.5 Oxygen Delivery Changes *34*
3.6 Conclusion *35*
References *35*

4 Macronutrients *39*
4.1 Introduction *39*
4.2 Carbohydrates *40*
4.2.1 Carbohydrates and Intensity *40*
4.2.2 Carbohydrate Structure and Metabolism *41*
4.2.3 Carbohydrate Deficiency and Performance *43*
4.2.4 The Glycemic Index *45*
4.2.5 Determining Carbohydrate Need *47*
4.3 Protein *49*
4.3.1 Assessing Protein Quality *50*
4.3.2 Nitrogen Balance *51*
4.3.3 Protein and Health *52*
4.3.4 Protein Requirements *53*
4.3.5 Protein Requirements for Older Athletes *55*
4.4 Fat (Lipids) *55*
4.4.1 Dietary Fat Classifications *56*
4.4.2 Fatty Acids *57*
4.4.3 Saturated or Unsaturated Fats *57*
4.4.4 Omega-3 and -6 Fatty Acids *58*
4.4.5 Essential Fatty Acids *58*

4.4.6	Ketogenic Diets and Performance *59*
4.5	Conclusion *60*
	References *61*

5 Micronutrients *63*
5.1	Introduction *63*
5.2	Vitamin Overview *63*
5.2.1	Water-Soluble Vitamins *64*
5.2.2	Fat-Soluble Vitamins *65*
5.2.3	Major Minerals *66*
5.2.4	Electrolytes *66*
5.2.5	Essential Trace Minerals *66*
5.2.6	Nonessential Trace Minerals *67*
5.3	Dietary Reference Intakes *67*
5.3.1	Limitations of the DRI *69*
5.3.2	Fortification vs Enrichment *70*
5.4	Water-Soluble Vitamins *70*
5.4.1	Vitamin B1 *71*
5.4.2	Vitamin B2 *72*
5.4.3	Vitamin B3 *72*
5.4.4	Vitamin B5 *73*
5.4.5	Vitamin B6 *74*
5.4.6	Vitamin B7 *75*
5.4.7	Folate *76*
5.4.8	Vitamin B12 *76*
5.4.9	Vitamin C *77*
5.5	Fat-Soluble Vitamins *78*
5.5.1	Vitamin A *78*
5.5.2	Vitamin D *79*
5.5.3	Vitamin K *80*
5.5.4	Vitamin E *81*
5.6	Electrolytes *82*
5.6.1	Sodium *82*
5.6.2	Chloride *82*
5.6.3	Potassium *83*
5.7	Major Minerals *83*
5.7.1	Calcium *83*
5.7.2	Phosphorus *84*
5.7.3	Magnesium *84*
5.8	Essential Trace Minerals *85*
5.8.1	Iron *85*

5.8.2   Zinc   86
5.8.3   Iodine   87
5.8.4   Selenium   88
5.8.5   Copper   88
5.8.6   Manganese   89
5.8.7   Chromium   90
5.8.8   Molybdenum   90
5.9   Nonessential Trace Minerals and Choline   91
5.9.1   Fluoride   91
5.9.2   Arsenic   91
5.9.3   Boron   91
5.9.4   Nickel   92
5.9.5   Silicon   92
5.9.6   Vanadium   93
5.9.7   Choline   93
5.10   Conclusion   94
         References   95

6   Nutrition Assessment   97
6.1   Introduction   97
6.2   Client History   97
6.3   Dietary Analysis   98
6.3.1   24-Hour Food Recall   99
6.3.2   Food Diaries   99
6.3.3   Food Frequency Questionnaire   101
6.3.4   When to Use Dietary Assessment Instruments   102
6.3.5   Indirect Calorimetry   103
6.4   Anthropometric Testing   104
6.4.1   Height   104
6.4.2   Weight   105
6.4.3   Body Measurements   105
6.4.4   Body Fat Measurements   107
6.4.5   Skinfold Caliper Measurements   107
6.4.6   Bioelectric Impedance Measurements   107
6.4.7   Hydrostatic Weighing   108
6.4.8   DEXA Body Fat Composition   108
6.4.9   Air Displacement Body Fat Composition   109
6.4.10   MRI and CT Body Fat Composition   109
6.5   Assessments of Hydration   109
6.5.1   Sweat Analysis   109
6.5.2   Sweat Rate Test   110

6.5.3	Sweat Sodium Concentration	*112*
6.5.4	Nonexercise Sweat Testing	*113*
6.6	Nutritionally Focused Lab Work	*114*
6.7	Conclusion	*115*
	References	*115*

7 Hydration *117*

7.1	Introduction	*117*
7.2	Water in the Body	*118*
7.3	Functions of Water	*118*
7.4	Sources of Water	*119*
7.5	Sources of Water Loss	*120*
7.6	Impact of Hydration Imbalance	*120*
7.7	Assessing Hydration Status	*121*
7.8	Hydration Strategies	*123*
7.9	Hydrating Sports Drinks	*125*
7.10	Conclusion	*126*
	References	*126*

8 Peri-workout Nutrition *129*

8.1	Introduction	*129*
8.2	Pre-workout Nutrition	*130*
8.2.1	Reactive Hypoglycemia	*131*
8.2.2	Carbohydrate Loading	*132*
8.3	Intra-workout Nutrition	*133*
8.4	Post-workout Nutrition	*134*
8.5	Conclusion	*135*
	References	*136*

9 Inflammation *139*

9.1	Introduction	*139*
9.2	The Physiology of Inflammation	*140*
9.2.1	Acute and Chronic Inflammation	*140*
9.3	Inflammation in Athletes	*141*
9.3.1	Exercise	*141*
9.3.2	Nutrition and Inflammation	*142*
9.3.3	Environment and Inflammation	*143*
9.4	Managing Inflammation for Performance	*143*
9.4.1	Dietary Strategies to Reduce Inflammation	*144*
9.4.1.1	Reduce Sources of Inflammation from the Diet	*144*
9.4.1.2	Increase the Consumption of Anti-inflammatory Foods	*144*

9.4.2	Supplementation to Reduce Inflammation	*146*
9.4.3	Recovery Techniques to Reduce Inflammation	*146*
9.5	Conclusion	*147*
	References	*147*

10 Supplementation *149*

10.1	Introduction	*149*
10.2	Supplementation vs Whole Foods	*150*
10.3	Muscle and Tissue Repair and Growth	*151*
10.3.1	Protein Powders	*152*
10.3.2	Amino Acid Supplementation	*155*
10.3.3	Branched Chain Amino Acids	*156*
10.3.4	Branched Chain Amino Acids vs Essential Amino Acids	*157*
10.3.5	Leucine	*158*
10.3.6	Ornithine	*158*
10.3.7	Glutamine	*159*
10.3.8	Beta-alanine	*160*
10.4	Carbohydrate Powders and Gels	*160*
10.5	Vitamins and Minerals	*162*
10.6	Oxidative Stress	*164*
10.6.1	*N*-Acetylcysteine	*164*
10.7	Hormone Balance and Cortisol Control	*165*
10.7.1	Dehydroepiandrostendione (DHEA)	*165*
10.7.2	Tribulus Terrestris	*167*
10.7.3	Phosphatidylserine	*167*
10.8	Inflammation Control	*168*
10.8.1	Fish Oil	*168*
10.8.2	Curcumin	*169*
10.8.3	Boswellia Serrata	*169*
10.8.4	Tart Cherry Juice	*170*
10.8.5	Quercetin	*170*
10.9	Ergogenic Supplements and Weight Loss	*170*
10.9.1	Creatine Monohydrate	*170*
10.9.2	Sodium Bicarbonate	*171*
10.9.3	Caffeine	*172*
10.9.4	Nitric Oxide	*174*
10.9.5	Chromium	*174*
10.9.6	Chitosan	*175*
10.9.7	Ephedrine	*175*
10.9.8	Pre-workout Supplementation	*176*
10.10	Microbiome Support	*176*

10.10.1	Probiotics	*177*
10.10.2	Prebiotic Supplements	*177*
10.11	Bone and Joint Support	*177*
10.11.1	Glucosamine	*177*
10.11.2	Chondroitin	*178*
10.11.3	Methylsulfonylmethane	*179*
10.12	Supplement Quality	*179*
10.13	Conclusion	*180*
	References	*181*
11	**Putting It All Together**	*191*
11.1	Introduction	*191*
11.2	Nutritional Assessment	*191*
11.2.1	Case Example	*192*
11.2.1.1	Significant History	*192*
11.2.1.2	Basic Anthropometric Measurements	*192*
11.2.1.3	Food Diary and FFQ Analysis	*192*
11.2.1.4	Macronutrient Averages	*192*
11.2.1.5	Current Supplements	*193*
11.2.1.6	Exercise Information	*193*
11.2.1.7	Initial Analysis	*193*
11.3	Establishing Dietary Goals	*193*
11.3.1	Case Example	*194*
11.4	Establishing Performance Metrics	*195*
11.4.1	Case Example	*196*
11.5	Creating the Nutritional Plan	*196*
11.6	Determining Caloric Needs	*197*
11.6.1	Total Caloric Requirements	*197*
11.6.2	Basal Metabolic Rate	*197*
11.6.3	The Thermic Effect of Activity	*199*
11.6.4	The Thermic Effect of Food	*199*
11.6.5	Determining the Basal Metabolic Rate	*200*
11.6.6	Activity Multiplier	*201*
11.6.7	Case Example	*202*
11.6.8	Alternate Methods for Calculation of Caloric Need	*202*
11.6.8.1	Cunningham Formula	*202*
11.6.8.2	Rule of Thumb	*203*
11.6.9	Case Example	*204*
11.7	Determination of Macronutrient Needs	*204*
11.7.1	Case Example	*204*
11.7.2	Case Example	*205*

11.8	Determination of Micronutrient Needs *206*
11.8.1	Case Example *206*
11.9	Developing a Hydration Strategy *206*
11.9.1	Case Example *207*
11.10	Establishing a Peri-workout Nutrition Plan *207*
11.10.1	Case Example *207*
11.11	Establishing a Targeted Supplementation Plan *208*
11.11.1	Case Example *208*
11.12	Conclusion *209*
	References *209*

Index *211*

Preface

The study of sports nutrition has been an important part of my career for the past 20 years. My introduction to sports nutrition began as my own Olympic aspirations as a weightlifter started to decline. In the late 1990s and early 2000s, I was a competitive Olympic-style weightlifter. I was able to compete at various local, regional, and national level events but aspired to earn a national team placement and even compete at an international competition. I may have been overestimating my abilities, but this was the driving force for my training during these years. At the time, I was competing in the superheavyweight division, weighing around 420 lbs. During my athletic career much of the nutritional information going around weightlifting circles was that to be able to compete as a drug-free athlete, you need to eat both a large amount of calories and protein. Supplements were discussed but discouraged for drug-tested athletes, due to the potential for adulteration. This made up the whole of my nutritional plan from the start of my career until around 2004. Around that time, as I approached 30 years old, I started to get nagging injuries which hurt my ability to train and compete. As a practicing chiropractor, with a focus on treating athletes, I had the knowledge and tools for the treatment and rehabilitation of these injuries but not enough information for their prevention from a nutritional perspective. I was personally using a mixture of chiropractic manipulation, rehabilitative exercise, massage, physical therapy, acupuncture, and various orthopedic injections to support my career. I would give myself rest and utilized various training and recovery modalities to support my performance but would find these injuries kept returning and amplifying. I was simply outperforming my ability to recover, and my body was paying the price in injuries. I finally realized that nutrition was a key piece of the performance puzzle that I had yet to explore. These injuries were not coming from breakdowns in technique, but rather a failure to match my diet to my training needs. I was not fueling recovery and performance adequately, and I was making poor food choices that limited my recovery and fueled the inflammatory process. I had been able to get away with eating pizza and fast food as a young athlete, but not any longer. Where previously I could recover from an extreme bout of exercise or small injury quickly, no matter what I ate, I now found that I was coming into workouts overtrained and achy. This epiphany led me to explore the world of sports nutrition. As a chiropractic student I had been exposed to a lot of quality nutrition education, but it focused mainly on general health. I could easily say that I had a good base of knowledge but needed more focused information in sports nutrition specifically. I then took it upon myself to read everything I could get my hands on both from popular media and peer-reviewed research. I took postgraduate educational courses and hired nutritionists to help me to learn. I found great success during this period of learning but felt a need to go deeper to understand how everything fit together. This led me to pursue a graduate education in nutrition.

My education and training provided me with the knowledge of how to put together an effective nutritional strategy for an athlete. I was able to create and oversee a nutritional plan that could support most athletes, but often found the needs of older athletes to be discussed as an afterthought or as a "special population." The reason for this, in my opinion, is that the nutritional needs of older athletes are not a seismic shift from those of a younger athlete. Instead, older athletes need a solid foundation of nutrition, similar to younger athletes, but with added focus of specific areas to adjust for the physiological impacts of aging and their impacts on recovery. This change, although seemingly small, has a lot to do with why implementing the nutritional strategies of younger athletes may look good but will not work as the athlete ages. The information was largely available, but not all in one place and rarely focused solely on older athletes.

Over the next 20 years of study, I have seen an evolution in the way that the subject of nutrition has been researched, specifically, as it applies to the needs of an older athlete. Unfortunately, while I have seen an increase in the knowledge base around older athletes, it was often difficult for me to find. I often had to rely on peer-reviewed research directly or through websites that often present incomplete or inaccurate information. This process of acquiring the knowledge to support an older athlete has been laborious and possibly is too cumbersome for many people who work with athletes. Coaches or healthcare professionals working with athletes may find it difficult to balance their direct work with athletes with all of the study needed for a strong evidence-based approach to sports nutrition for masters athletes.

I am still very active in athletics and still train to about 70–80% of my younger intensity while weighing about 60–70% of my competitive bodyweight. Through the methods contained in this book, I have been able to maintain a lot of my younger performance while reducing the long-term health risks I faced in my early thirties. In many ways, I feel more capable at 48 than I did at 38; this is due to the application of many of the strategies contained in this book. I still get injuries and bouts of overtraining, but I am better able to recover from them and perform. I plan to maintain this level of training for as long as possible to maintain a full and active life.

Unfortunately, the development of this knowledge has taken two decades of work and come too late for my Olympic dreams. Thankfully this information can be used by nutritional providers as a roadmap to help other aging athletes to achieve their goals. As the participation in sports by older athletes increases, there is a need to provide those who work with athletes over the age of 35 a handbook that they can follow from start to finish without having to sift through nutritional protocols and strategies that do not relate to this specific demographic. The goal of this book was to assemble the key elements of sports nutrition, as they affect older athletes, into one place to be used as a resource for those who work with older athletes, or for the athletes themselves. Please use the information contained within this book to assist the athletes you work with to achieve their performance goals whatever they may be.

1

Overview

1.1 Introduction

The impact of sports nutrition on an athlete's performance has been well-established. Sports nutrition is an important part of the athlete's training and recovery regime. Sports nutrition serves two separate but important roles for the athlete. The first role of sports nutrition is to provide the fuel for how we participate in or train for athletic events. Macronutrients in the form of carbohydrates, proteins, and fats provide the athlete with the energy needed to fuel athletic training and competition, and the micronutrients consisting of vitamins and minerals are needed for their coenzyme and cofactor roles in assisting to fuel these activities. This role of sports nutrition is well-established and relatively stable across different age strata. Athletes of all ages and capabilities will need to use nutrition to fuel their athletic endeavors. The second role of nutrition for an athlete has more to do with recovery from exercise and the rebuilding of muscle tissues following exercise. This role is also well-established, but is more intricate and will require a more specialized approach where the athlete's individual nutritional needs to be able to recover and rebuild should be accounted for. The nutritional needs of an athlete will differ depending on the specific sport involved, the type of training, and some specific factors related to the individual athlete. The needs of a 55-year-old athlete to recover from a weight training session, for example, are not the same as the nutritional needs of an 18-year-old athlete doing the same activity, much like the nutritional needs of a male and female athlete in the same sport are not the same. This book will focus on the specific nutritional needs of athletes over the age of 35 as they seek to train and compete in sports. This group of athletes must balance

Sports Nutrition for Masters Athletes, First Edition. Peter G. Nickless.
© 2025 John Wiley & Sons, Inc. Published 2025 by John Wiley & Sons, Inc.

their nutritional needs with ever-changing physiological characteristics that impact their ability to recover and perform in their chosen sport. It is through an understanding of the nutritional needs of an athlete for them to be able to train and compete in their sport, knowledge of the physiologic changes associated with the aging process, and the creation of nutrition and supplemental strategies to mitigate some of these effects that someone who works with older athletes can best be able to support their performance. These are the topics that this book seeks to address. The contents of this book will assist the nutritional professional looking to work with a master's athlete or the athlete themselves to optimize nutritional approaches to positively impact their athlete's performance while reducing the overall impact of these physiologic changes associated with aging.

1.2 Demographic Data

Athletic participation by older individuals is growing at a rapid pace. The 35+ age demographic is currently a rapidly growing segment of the population, as well as the competitive athletic market. Advances in nutrition, sports science, and healthcare have allowed athletes to train and perform at older ages than ever possible. Adding to this increased awareness of the impact of exercise and activity on longevity and mobility, we see an increase in athletic participation in this age group growing rapidly. The increase in athletic participation is fueled by the reduced attrition of younger athletes as they age, keeping them in the competition pool longer, and the increase in new athletes who take up a sport at an older age. In the sport of Olympic-style weightlifting, for example, we have seen a nearly threefold increase in the number of competitors at the masters (over 35 years old) age division national championship, with 244 athletes competing in 2015 to 718 athletes competing in 2019. The largest increase was seen in the number of female competitors, who went from 44.4% of all competitors to 58.7% [1]. This desire to train and compete in older age groups presents an interesting opportunity for those working with athletes. An older athletic population has some beneficial aspects: they tend to have both more time and money for training and nutrition. Both factors represent significant barriers to training and competition for younger athletes. Unfortunately, there is also an increase in the likelihood of injuries associated with their athletic participation. This is where the field of sports nutrition can have an impact [1, 2].

1.3 What Is Sports Nutrition?

Sports nutrition is a specialized focus area of the research and clinical field of nutrition. This field of study looks at the physiologic function of the human body in various exercise-related areas and the role that nutrients and hydration may have in impacting these processes. Sports nutrition is where the fields of physiology, exercise science, and human nutrition meet to impact athletic performance and recovery. The key objective of sports nutrition is to improve athletic performance and increase the longevity of the athlete in their sport. Although sports nutrition is often associated with high-level athletes like Olympians, professional bodybuilders, or professional athletes, this field of study is not reserved for elite athletes only but rather for anyone looking to improve their performance in their chosen athletic endeavor. Sports nutrition is focused on the nutrients needed to support the body's recovery and repair processes and is an extension of traditional nutrition. Many of the principles of sports nutrition match those for general health, but there are differences in the quantity and timing of nutrients. The nutrients needed by the athlete vary more in amount than the type compared to the needs of the general public, for the most part. Still, often, the need to meet the increased requirements of an athlete looking to perform their best makes dietary planning and supplementation more of a necessity.

1.4 Why Study Sports Nutrition?

Sports nutrition is an important field of study for athletes, nutritionists, coaches, and anybody interested in achieving optimal sports performance. The physical aspect of training represents an essential element of athletic performance. The athlete's training program today can significantly impact future performance, but this is not the only crucial factor the athlete needs to consider [3]. Other factors such as nutrition, rest, technique, equipment, or even psychological state will all play their role in an athlete's overall performance. For anybody working with athletes, addressing the nutritional plan must be considered an important element in performance and be treated as an essential factor in the athlete's performance plan. Sports nutrition can impact recovery from exercise, tissue rebuilding, the control of the inflammatory process and response, and can even impact the general health of the athlete. Therefore, anyone looking to achieve maximal performance in an athletic event will need to factor an individualized nutritional strategy into their training regime. While primarily focused on athletes, the author would contend that the study of sports nutrition dives into the physiologic functions regarding the utilization of energy optimally by the body. Studying the material contained within this book will carry relevance to everyone, regardless of athletic capabilities.

1.5 What Is a Masters Athlete?

Athletes come in all shapes and sizes. This feature of athletics is what allows for so many people to compete because there is no standard "athlete" in regard to this aspect. We have small athletes who compete in events based on power-to-weight ratio, such as in sports like rock climbing. We have larger athletes competing in sports such as professional football, where absolute power and speed are more important, and every type of athlete in between. Athletes can also be found in differing sexes, each with unique nutritional requirements. Additionally, we find athletes in a wide spectrum of ages with youth sports, sometimes starting sports as early as three years old, all the way up to geriatric athletic participants. Sports will often stratify athlete competitions based on many of these categories. Sports, both at the local and national level, can carry age divisions such as youth, junior, senior, and masters athletes. In the sport of weightlifting, for example, youth athletes compete from 13 years old up to 17 years of age. Junior athletes will compete in their age group from 18 to 23 years old. The term senior athlete is typically associated with an athlete in the 24- to 34-year-old age group (this can get confusing as in the general population, the term senior is often associated with older adults). The term master's athlete is a designation given to athletes competing at the age of 35 and over. There are some variations in these age ranges in other sports, as individual sports organizations will vary in their competitive age categories, but generally, these categories will remain similar. The contents of this book will cover the physiologic and nutritional needs that will impact athletes of all ages but are specifically targeted at master's age group athletes 35 and over.

1.6 Why Focus on Masters Athletes?

There are numerous intelligent reasons to focus on a population like master's athletes, not the least of which is that they represent a large, growing sector of the athletic population. This population sector is growing but has either been treated as an afterthought or marginalized by much of the community. Sports nutrition texts, for the most part, focus on athletes in their teens through their early 40s. There are chapters and articles focused on older athletes, but not many entire books. In the past 20 years, one of the largest growth sectors in athletic events and training has been in athletes ages 35 and up [1, 2]. This means that a significant portion of the athletic community often gets reduced to a chapter or section of a chapter in a traditional sports nutrition book. Unfortunately, these athletes do not recover the same way as younger athletes. These changes impact the athlete's recovery, rebuilding, and performance, which will lead to significantly differing nutritional requirements compared to the needs of a 17-year-old or even a 30-year-old athlete. While there are many similarities between athletes in all age ranges, there are also needs for fueling performance and recovery that are significantly different for older athletes. Differences in macro- and micronutrient needs, hydration requirements, and supplement recommendations necessitate a deeper focus on this athletic population. Accordingly, it is both the size of the master's athletic population combined with their specific nutritional needs that make this age demographic a segment of the athletic population that should be examined further. This book seeks to fill this gap by addressing the nutritional needs of older athletes as they seem to optimize their performance and recovery.

1.7 What Are the Nutrients Used by Athletes?

The link between nutrition and sports performance is well-established. While it is understood by many that nutrition is an important consideration for athletes, of all ages, the actual nutrients that the athlete will need and when they will need them are much less understood. This lack of knowledge can lead to miscommunication in the world of sports nutrition. This results in athletes not getting all the benefits of a well-designed nutritional strategy. One example of this is the general understanding that any athlete looking to put on muscle needs to eat protein. This is true in general but fails to consider the nutritional needs to digest the protein, the other macronutrients needed to help support muscle growth, and the nutrients that may help the athlete perform their training to the highest degree to allow for muscle growth. In this respect simply eating more protein is only one small piece of the sports nutrition strategy. The ubiquitous nature of supplementation in sports nutrition can amplify this concern. Sports supplementation is everywhere, and many supplement advertisements tend to advocate individual nutrients as the "key" to unlocking sports performance potential. Drinks, shakes, bars, powders, and pills are marketed for their ability to potentially help the athlete to perform at their best, but it is less common to hear about the role of supplements as part of a well-designed nutritional strategy to improve performance. The reality is that the sports nutritional palate is diverse and must be examined collectively. This is not to say that there are no supplements that can directly impact performance, but rather, they must be taken within the context of a well-planned nutritional strategy. Therefore, any book focusing on the clinical application of nutrition for older athletes should first define the nutrients the athlete needs to be able to perform.

1.8 Macronutrients

The first classification of nutrients needed for optimal performance is the Macronutrients. Macronutrients provide the athlete energy from calories, including carbohydrates, lipids (or fats), and protein. This classification of nutrients carries the term "Macro" because they are needed in larger quantities. These nutrients make up the backbone of a sound nutritional plan. These nutrients can come to the diet from both plant and animal sources. Carbohydrates provide the body, among other things, with the energy needed to perform physical activities. Fiber is a specific carbohydrate category with crucial physiological functions, and is vital to the athlete's health, and plays an important role in blood sugar regulation but does not directly provide the body with energy for athletic performance. Lipids also have many roles among them: energy storage, the synthesis of hormones, the absorption and storage of fat-soluble vitamins, and aiding in nerve conduction, for example, through myelination. Proteins serve both structural and functional roles physiologically. Structurally, protein is needed for the growth and development of muscles and the recovery from exercise. Functionally, proteins can act as, among other things, enzymes needed to initiate physiologic reactions. Together, these nutrients comprise the majority of the diet and define the caloric make-up of the athlete's nutritional plan. We will explore each of these in more detail in Chapter 4.

1.9 Micronutrients

The next classification of nutrients we will discuss is the micronutrients. These nutrients are used by the body to support normal physiological functions along with the macronutrients. The term "micronutrients" is derived from the fact that they are needed in a lower volume for use in the body.

Micronutrients can be subdivided into vitamins, minerals, and elements. Many of these vitamins, minerals, and elements are essential to many physiologic processes and are required from the diet. This classification of nutrients does not contain any calories themselves or directly provide the body with energy. Still, they are important in their use as cofactors in the processes where the body derives energy from macronutrients, such as the biochemical process of glycolysis. All these micronutrients carry some function, and most are needed to some degree to assist the body in maintaining health and have roles in athletic performance, although the type and amount will differ for athletes, particularly masters athletes. This topic will be addressed in more detail in Chapter 5 of this book.

1.10 Hydration

Water is essential to maintaining physiological processes. Approximately 70% of the human body is made up of water. Water, whether from consumption or internal production, is important as both a reactant and byproduct of the body's chemical reactions. Accordingly, the balance of water in the body is a critical factor in supporting physiological functions and optimal athletic performance and recovery. There is a direct relationship between hydration and performance, and poor hydration is linked to decreased athletic performance [4]. This carries a particular relevance for the older athlete, who carries a greater risk for dehydration when compared to their younger counterparts. The assessment of hydration and the development of a hydration plan to fuel performance and prevent dehydration will be discussed further in Chapter 7.

1.11 Supplementation

The final element of a nutritional plan that will be discussed will be supplementation. Supplementation refers to the nutritional aids that are used to support the diet to correct any nutritional shortcomings or to enhance performance and recovery. The first of these items, correcting nutritional shortcomings, can also impact performance if the nutrient needed for supplementation is deficient. However, supplementing deficient nutrients does not always translate to improved performance beyond correcting the nutritional deficiency. The second role of a supplement can be those that are used to improve performance by adding specific nutrients that have a known benefit to athletes extending beyond the correction of a deficiency.

An example of this is caffeine, which can have the potential to improve athletic performance for the athlete but is not given to correct any deficiency. Issues with supplementation involve potential toxicities from their use and, more commonly, overuse. The quality and source of the supplement are also a concern, as the effects of the supplement may be limited or altered due to poor quality or adulterated products. Overall, supplementation can be an important element of the nutritional programming for a master's athlete. The topic of supplementation will be discussed in more depth in Chapter 10.

1.12 Overview: A Nutrient Approach to Diet

Now that we have discussed an overview of the nutritional elements that make up an athlete's performance plan, it is important to give a general overview of how to put it all together. This leads to the question of how we combine all these nutrients to develop a strong nutritional strategy for the athlete. While we will go deeper into this subject in Chapter 11, let us examine an overall structure for our approach. An important consideration in determining nutritional needs for athletes, regardless of age, is a hierarchical structure. This means those working with athletes need to look at the nutrient decisions in the context of how they relate to each other in order of importance from the most important to the least important. This allows the practitioner or coach to prioritize their approach and refine results as they go, with all other recommendations under consideration. If visualized, this structure should resemble a flow chart with the progress of the nutritional evaluation moving from the bottom to the top. The flow chart is a good way to think of it as the bottom is the starting point from which all other nutritional considerations start acting as a base or foundation. From there, we move up the chart, with each step building on the previous one. Nutritionally, we start with the most important nutritional factor and then work toward the overall goal. Moving further up the flow chart, we see further delineations that are less important, than the base, but still vital to hitting peak performance (Figure 1.1).

When working with athletes, I always recommend starting with a conversation about goals. It is important, when working with an athlete nutritionally, that we can determine what the athlete is looking to accomplish, both with the presenting proposed dietary changes and from their athletic career in general. For example, a sports nutritionist or anyone working with a sports nutrition client may have some ideas to improve an athlete's performance. Based on their initial presentation and where the practitioner wants to see the athlete's career progress, however, this may not coincide with the athlete's goals. For example, if, despite the thoughts of the nutrition professional, the athlete is looking to optimize performance while dropping down a weight class, there is likely going to be an issue if the weight loss limits performance, as is the case with many sports. There may be a mismatch between the plans or ideas of the nutrition professional and the athlete, and we need to know from the start if that athlete can achieve maximal performance based on their goals. If there is a mismatch between the nutritional practitioner and the athlete's goals, adjustments should be made to accommodate the athlete's personal or performance goals. The athlete's goals will always be paramount to those of the nutrition professional and will need to be considered when determining any nutritional plans. Accordingly, every conversation about sports nutrition must clarify the athlete's goals. Once these goals are established, the coach or nutritional professional has a desired outcome to which the diet can be tailored.

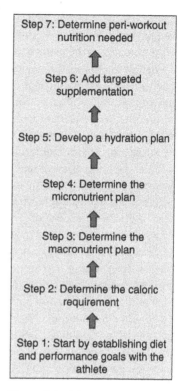

Figure 1.1 Hierarchy of the determination of nutritional needs.

Our next step up the flow chart is to look at the caloric requirements for the athlete to meet their goals. Recently, there has been some debate about whether calories should be the most important factor in sports nutrition, and some will focus straight away on the macronutrient needs. This would be a mistake as caloric requirements serve as an important base and starting point when examining the dietary needs of any athlete. It would be difficult, although not impossible, to accurately determine a macronutrient plan without knowing the intended overall calories the athlete will need. The caloric requirements of each athlete should be personalized and need to consider factors such as the age, the sex of the athlete, and the athlete's weight. The athlete's goals should also be considered when determining caloric requirements as well. For example, if weight gain, weight loss, or weight maintenance are important, alterations from the base caloric requirement must be made to accommodate these goals.

After determining the caloric needs of the athlete, the next step is to determine the macronutrient breakdown in a manner that will enable the athlete to be able to fuel performance. There are several methods of determining the macronutrient distribution which remain to be discussed later in this book. Still, determining the macronutrient plan needs to start with an emphasis on the requirements and demands of the individual sport being trained for or contested. Each sport will have different physiologic demands and will determine the macronutrient ratios required to optimize performance. For example, an endurance-based athlete will not necessarily need the same number of grams of carbohydrates as a strength-based athlete, as the demands of long-duration endurance exercise demand a lot more fuel from carbohydrates to perform the activity.

After determining macronutrient requirements, the coach or nutrition professional should examine the micronutrient needs, which will differ for each athlete as the vitamin and mineral needs will alter somewhat through aging. After considering calories, macro, and micronutrients, the coach or nutritional professional should focus on hydration, as dehydration can lead to decreased athletic performance or even a potential injury. We consider supplementation only after considering all these previous factors. Supplementation is an important factor; not every athlete will need or should include supplementation. Supplementation should be personalized and have a performance or health-related purpose. This supplementation should be targeted and evidence-based to assist the athlete in achieving their athletic goals but should be secondary to dietary efforts. Finally, peri-workout nutrition should be planned both for training periods as well as during competition. Peri-workout nutrition is the food and supplements consumed before, during, or right after training or competition that are targeted at fueling performance and recovery. This could be considered to be the pinnacle of the chart as it takes the determination of all of the other elements prior to truly developing a solid peri-workout nutritional plan.

1.13 Conclusion

This book will be a clinical handbook for those who wish to work with older athletes or for the athletes themselves as they seek to find the method to best fuel optimal athletic performance. The reader, be they professional nutritionist, doctor, coach, or athlete, should be able to use the information gained from reading this book to better assist athletes over the age of 35 to develop the nutritional strategy that will fuel optimal performance and recovery. The contents of this book represent the current state of nutritional information with a focus on clinical application. This means the author's goal is for the information presented to be used rather than simply learned. The information in this book is by no means a complete representation of the sports nutrition field overall nor a substitute for medical advice. Just as individuals come in all shapes and sizes, they also come with a variety of pre-existing conditions that must be considered by those working with them. The information gained in the book should be used to aid those working with athletes but not taken as a direct prescription.

References

1 Huebner M, Meltzer D, Ma W, Arrow H. The Masters athlete in Olympic weightlifting: training, lifestyle, health challenges, and gender differences [published correction appears in PLoS One. 2021 Feb 10;16(2):e0247110]. *PLoS One* 2020;15(12):e0243652. Published 2020 Dec 4. doi:10.1371/journal.pone.0243652

2 Jenkin CR, Eime RM, Westerbeek H, O'Sullivan G, van Uffelen JGZ. Sport and ageing: a systematic review of the determinants and trends of participation in sport for older adults. *BMC Public Health* 2017;17(1):976. Published 2017 Dec 22. doi:10.1186/s12889-017-4970-8

3 Malsagova KA, Kopylov AT, Sinitsyna AA, et al. Sports nutrition: diets, selection factors, recommendations. *Nutrients* 2021;13(11):3771. Published 2021 Oct 25. doi:10.3390/nu13113771

4 Maughan RJ, Shirreffs SM. Nutrition for sports performance: issues and opportunities. *Proc. Nutr. Soc.* 2012;71(1):112–119. doi:10.1017/S0029665111003211

2

A Biochemistry and Physiology

2.1 Introduction

An examination of the role of nutrition can have on athletic performance first requires a discussion of the underlying biochemical and physiological processes involved with the metabolism of food and nutrient use in the body. A more thorough understanding of these physiological processes, by which we turn nutrients into the substrate needed to fuel performance or support recovery, will enhance our understanding of the purpose of the nutritional plans we seek to design and allow the practitioner to be able to design a more effective strategy. In addition to the underlying biochemistry, we also need a basic understanding of some principles of exercise physiology and how this relates to how these principles may differ based on the specific athletic events or training we are trying to fuel. It is essential that anyone working with athletes learn about the individual sports being trained for and contested. The nutritional professional must understand the specifics of the athletic event, the intensity of the event, the training involved, and the duration of the event, both in training and competition, to guide their nutritional plan to feed the needs of the athlete. Let us look at the energy systems used in sports; for example, understanding the different energy systems used in sports and the nutrients used to fuel those energy systems can help to target an appropriate nutritional strategy. The goal, for the nutritional professional, is to understand the energy systems and underlying physiology well enough to be able to match the diet strategy to the needs of the athlete's chosen athletic event. If the athlete, for example, were operating primarily in shorter-duration sports, this would point us in the direction of the type of nutrients we need to include in the plan. On the other hand,

Sports Nutrition for Masters Athletes, First Edition. Peter G. Nickless.
© 2025 John Wiley & Sons, Inc. Published 2025 by John Wiley & Sons, Inc.

setting up a diet loaded with fuel sources for longer-duration energy systems may be better for someone who trains and competes in longer-duration events like a marathon. This chapter will explore the physiology involved in the metabolism of nutrients and the energy systems used in sports. The goal here is not an encyclopedic understanding of the subject but a working knowledge a practitioner can use to directly impact the performance of an athlete.

2.2 Homeostasis

One overarching principle that is essential to the understanding of how physiological processes work is homeostasis. Homeostasis refers to the state of physiologic balance where the body is neither building new tissue nor fighting disease. In other words, this is a state of equilibrium in which the body functions healthily through the harmonious interplay between organ systems. An example of this is how the body maintains blood sugar within a specific range. If someone were to eat too much sugar, assuming no pathological condition exists, the body would recognize this and release insulin from the beta cells of the pancreas to remove excess sugar from the blood to be stored in the muscles and liver as glycogen. If the body experiences a reduction in blood sugar, on the other hand, the hormone glucagon is released from the alpha cells of the pancreas to remove the stored glycogen to be broken down thereby increasing the blood sugar. This relationship between the hormones insulin and glucagon is essential for maintaining homeostatic balance. Typically, homeostatic balance is maintained using feedback loops. Two types of feedback loops are employed by the body to maintain equilibrium. The positive feedback loop is one where the stimulus received will trigger a stronger response, which in turn will stimulate another response, etc. This feedback loop usually needs a major event to stop it from continuing. A typical example of this would be labor in childbirth. In this case, the uterine contraction, brought on by the hormone oxytocin, stimulates the next uterine contraction. This will continue and intensify until the child is born, stopping the continuation of the feedback loop. The more common feedback loop experienced in the body would be a negative feedback loop. In a negative feedback loop, the stimulus initiates a response to counteract the stimulus. Unlike with a positive feedback loop, the response to the stimulus stops as soon as the desired outcome is achieved. The example above with insulin is a great example of a negative feedback loop. The stimulus of elevated blood sugar leads to the response of insulin secretion to lower the blood sugar. As the blood sugar returns to normal limits, insulin secretion is stopped. In this case, the term negative is used because the response would be stopped once the stimulus is removed. As we can see, the body uses these feedback loops to help maintain homeostatic balance and, by extension, health. Homeostasis plays an important role in the biochemistry of an athlete as the athlete provides stimulus to the body in the form of activity. The body needs to respond to this activity by providing the energy to perform activities, regulating the activities performed, and recovering and rebuilding from the activity. In this case, homeostasis is lost as soon as the demands on the body exceed the current state of physiological activity. This requires the athlete to react to the stimulus by increasing physiological processes to meet the new demand and regain homeostasis. If we limit our discussion to just energy, for example, the body must release stored energy from glycogen and create new energy through a process called glycolysis. These systems provide the athlete with energy to perform their activities and are discontinued when the athlete no longer needs energy. In this way, a negative feedback loop is being used to help the athlete maintain homeostatic balance.

2.3 Energy Production

Athletic performance at a biochemical level is focused, in part, on the production, storage, and utilization of energy. Energy is needed to, among other things, drive the muscles, move blood through vessels, and fuel the brain to be able to perform an athletic activity. Energy, specifically the production of energy, is a key goal of sports nutrition practitioners. We can achieve optimal performance through understanding and effectively utilizing the processes of energy production. If the athlete is provided enough energy, they can perform to their maximal capabilities, but if they are provided too little energy, athletic performance will decline as the body is forced to use stored energy from body fat or, to a lesser extent, break down muscle to maintain energy homeostasis. On the other hand, if too much energy is available beyond the requirements of the athlete, the body will store the excess energy as glycogen and body fat. This can be a more long-term problem for performance as excess body fat accumulation can interfere with athletic performance for some sports and in the long-term excess body fat can carry health implications through associations with many chronic diseases such as diabetes and heart disease. As nutritional practitioners, we must seek a balance between the energy the athlete provides and their performance requirements based on the activity. In other words, we must find the exact point of energy homeostasis.

The energy needed to fuel athletic activity comes either directly from the dietary macronutrients carbohydrates, fats, and protein or from stored energy in the form of body fat. Energy consumed from macronutrients comes in the form of calories. A calorie is a measurement that represents a unit of energy. It is calculated as the amount of heat energy required to raise the temperature of 1 g of water by 1 °C. All calories consumed must be digested, absorbed, and metabolized for use at the cellular level or stored for later use. The biochemical processes of the metabolism of these nutrients and stored body fat produce a chemical called adenosine triphosphate (ATP). This chemical is a form of cellular energy that can be synthesized by the various biochemical pathways in which we metabolize dietary macronutrients.

2.3.1 Forms of Energy

ATP is the storage form of energy in the human body at the cellular level. The ATP molecule consists of an adenine base and a ribose sugar attached to three phosphate groups. Energy is released to fuel cellular metabolism when breaking a chemical bond removes one of the three phosphate groups. The breaking of the chemical bond with one of the three phosphate groups creates adenosine diphosphate or ADP. ADP is like ATP, a stored form of energy. We have the same chemical composition of one adenine base with a ribose sugar, but only two phosphate groups are attached. Functionally, ADP is seen as the byproduct of converting ATP from stored to kinetic energy. Although further removing a phosphate group would produce more energy from the breakdown of the chemical bond producing adenosine monophosphate or AMP, the more efficient use is adding a phosphate group to produce ATP for physiological use. AMP is a nucleotide in the body consisting of an adenosine base, a ribose sugar, and a single phosphate group. AMP is used for various physiologic purposes in the body but is also used for the conversion process to ADP and then ATP for use as an energy source to fuel athletic performance. For the purpose of this book, the biochemical processes we will be discussing involve producing energy in the form of ATP by adding a phosphate group to the ADP molecule.

2.4 Biochemical Reactions in Sports Nutrition

Metabolism refers to the various biochemical reactions by which the body converts various reactants into energy to satisfy physiological needs. In sports nutrition, metabolism typically focuses on the biochemical pathways by which energy, in the form of ATP, is produced from macronutrients. Other examples of metabolic processes involve the synthesis of glycogen, the synthesis of amino acids, or fatty acids. Examples of the actual metabolic processes would include glycolysis (which converts glucose to pyruvic acid, which then can enter the tricarboxylic acid cycle) and ketogenesis (which can convert fatty acids into ketone bodies for use by the tricarboxylic acid cycle to produce ATP).

2.4.1 Glycolysis

Glycolysis, or the glycolytic pathway, is the most important and most commonly referred to biochemical processes in sports nutrition. At its most basic, glycolysis is the process in which the monosaccharide (to be discussed in Chapter 4 with macronutrients) glucose can be broken down into two pyruvic acid molecules. In addition to the two pyruvic acid molecules, a small amount of ATP molecules are produced. The pyruvic acid, in the absence of oxygen, is converted to lactic acid. This process is called anaerobic glycolysis. If oxygen is present, the pyruvate molecules can be converted to acetyl-CoA, which can be used in the tricarboxylic acid cycle to produce even more energy [1].

2.4.2 Beta-oxidation

Beta-oxidation refers to the biochemical process by which fatty acids can be converted to energy for use. In this process, free fatty acids, formed from the metabolism of dietary fat, are converted to acetyl-CoA for further use in the tricarboxylic acid cycle for the production of energy. It is through the beta-oxidation cycle that the athlete is able to use fatty acids, derived from either the diet or from the breakdown of body fat, to supply the energy production needs of the body [1].

2.4.3 Gluconeogenesis

Gluconeogenesis is the process by which glucose can be produced from noncarbohydrates. This process involves essentially the glycolysis process in reverse from pyruvate to glucose. The precursors that can be used for gluconeogenesis include glycerol from fatty acids, lactate, pyruvate, and some amino acids. Gluconeogenesis comes into play in a starvation state, either from fasting, inadequate nutrition, or starvation as the body starts to need glucose for the maintenance of homeostatic balance [1].

2.4.4 Tricarboxylic Acid Cycle

The tricarboxylic acid cycle or Krebs cycle is the biochemical process by which acetyl-CoA is converted into energy for use by athletes. The acetyl-CoA is derived from carbohydrates, fats, and proteins through various biochemical processes. It is through these processes that we can derive the majority of the substrate needed to produce the large amount of energy needed for various athletic purposes. This process is oxygen-dependent and results in significantly more ATP production when compared to glycolysis alone [1].

2.4.5 Ketogenesis

If energy is not needed, the acetyl-CoA can be converted to ketone bodies using ketogenesis. Ketogenesis refers to the process by which acetyl-CoA can be converted to the three ketone bodies: acetone, acetoacetate, and beta-hydroxybutyrate. Ketogenesis is stimulated by starvation, a low carbohydrate diet, and prolonged exercise. These ketone bodies can be reconverted to acetyl-CoA to make energy through the tricarboxylic acid cycle [1].

2.4.6 Glycogenesis

Glycogenesis is the biochemical process by which excess carbohydrates are stored in the liver and muscle as glycogen. This process is activated by insulin as a reaction to elevated blood sugar. Glycogenesis and glycogenolysis work together to maintain homeostasis in relation to blood sugar [1].

2.4.7 Glycogenolysis

Glycogenolysis occurs in the skeletal muscle and the liver, where stored glucose in the form of glycogen is released and converted back to glucose for use. Glycogenolysis is stimulated by the hormone glucagon. This process can provide a fast source of energy for muscles to use and comes into play during states of fasting, starvation, or inadequate nutrition to fuel activities. The process of glycogenolysis is quicker than gluconeogenesis, but there are more limitations as the body can only produce glucose in relation to the amount of stored glycogen. Gluconeogenesis, while less efficient, has less limitation in substrate [1].

Anabolism refers to the metabolic processes by which the body converts smaller molecules into larger ones. Typically, in sports nutrition, this will refer to "building" type reactions. For example, protein assists in building muscle with training, so protein participates in an anabolic process.

Catabolism refers to the biochemical properties by which more complex molecules are broken down into smaller, simpler molecules. In sports nutrition, we typically refer to catabolic processes as those that break down nutrients into smaller ones for use. For example, dietary protein must be broken down into individual amino acids for use by biochemical processes. Catabolism and anabolism will often work together.

2.5 Energy Systems

Although the focus of this book is sports nutrition, the aim of any well-constructed nutritional plan needs to include knowledge of the individual sport or sports being trained for and contested by the athlete. This puts pressure on the nutritional professional to learn at least a little about exercise physiology, or at least some of the specific elements of exercise physiology, and the specific energy demands of some individual sports. An examination of the energy systems used by sports to fuel optimal performance will help the nutritional practitioner or coach to better target a nutrition plan to the athlete's needs. The reason to understand energy systems and how they are associated with individual sports is that there needs to be a solid understanding of the demands placed on the athlete. These demands may differ based on either the individual sport being contested or the phase of training for the athlete. For example, a hockey player will have a practice consisting of about one hour of intense training with several stops and starts. This more likely resembles the high-intensity training of a sprinter. An ultra runner, on the other hand, may have workouts that consist of longer duration runs that may last up to several hours. The activity will not be as intense in terms of their VO_2 max or the heart rate elevation for the runner will not raise as high as the hockey player's does. The two examples require the same nutrients but in different ratios and amounts so that they can supply the differing energy systems used with the appropriate nutrients needed as fuel. An additional benefit of examining the energy systems used in a particular sport is that it is an excellent opportunity to connect with the athlete and form a relationship. Once the athlete realizes that that you have taken the time to understand their needs based on their athletic schedule, it should help to develop trust and get a greater "buy-in" from your athlete, and hopefully, better adherence to the nutritional strategy. An important part of truly understanding individuals' nutritional needs is a thorough examination of the energy systems required to perform their chosen sport at given stages of training. This will be true of athletes of all ages, although physiologic adaptations due to age must be considered.

2.5.1 What Are Energy Systems?

The food we eat and, to a lesser extent, the supplements we take serve as the source of energy to meet the requirements to perform athletic activity. We take in nutrients in the form of carbohydrates, fats, and proteins to fuel athletic performance, but how they do it and in what ratio differs based on the energy systems involved. Although we use food and supplements to meet our energy requirements, the nutrients must first be metabolized and converted to a form usable by the body. To supply the body's energy needs and avoid ATP fatigue, the nutrients must be converted to ATP, the usable form of energy for the body. ATP fatigue in exercise refers to when the work output required cannot be maintained by the energy production available to the athlete. This means that the athlete will no longer be able to provide nutrients and oxygen to the tissues to support athletic performance. One reason for this fatigue is that the exercise intensity of the sport in question is so high that it outpaces the ATP production available to meet the performance demand [2]. This scenario is typically seen in short-duration, high-intensity sports such as sprinting or a fast-paced shift in ice hockey.

As stated, the process by which nutrients are converted to ATP is called an energy system. There are three energy systems utilized in the human body. We have the phosphagen system, which supplies our immediate energy needs. Anaerobic glycolysis provides fuel for short-term activities. Finally, we have aerobic glycolysis, which is much slower and uses either carbohydrates, fats, or, in some cases, proteins to help supply us with energy for longer-duration activities. It is important to note that for many athletic activities, all three energy systems will be used to fuel performance, the degree to which will differ depending on the sport or training phase [3]. Additionally, the ratios of nutrients needed to fuel these energy systems will change based on differing activities and must be considered.

2.5.2 Phosphagen System

As previously mentioned, the energy needs for the performance of an athlete can be satisfied using ATP. Initially, this ATP can be found freely circulating in the bloodstream, but it only takes a few seconds before it is depleted and will need replenishment. After this free circulating ATP is used, the athlete must rapidly produce new ATP from ADP. This is commonly done by adding a phosphate group ADP, converting it to ATP for use by the body. This will allow the athlete to continue to fuel athletic activity while using ATP. The phosphagen system is the energy system used to convert ADP to ATP. This system requires circulating creatine phosphate and ADP.

Creatine phosphate is found in about four to five times greater concentration than circulating ATP, and the phosphagen system can supply enough ATP to fuel about 12–30 seconds of activity. The phosphagen system, of course, will be the primary source of energy for initiating athletic activity and a leading energy source for skill-based or extremely short-duration activities. The athlete can expect a 50% recovery following 30 seconds of rest or 100% recovery after 2 minutes. If we were to look at a competitive weightlifting event where we would see a single lift at near maximal exertion followed by a period of rest before the next attempt, this would be an ideal energy system to fuel this activity. Extension of the activity beyond this short 30-second period, without rest, will require additional energy systems.

2.5.3 Anaerobic Glycolysis

The process of metabolizing nutrients, most commonly glucose, for energy is called glycolysis. Glycolysis, as explained earlier in this chapter, is the metabolic pathway associated with energy production and can be further differentiated between aerobic glycolysis and aerobic glycolysis. Anaerobic glycolysis will be utilized primarily following the initial 30-second phase of the phosphagen system as the need for ATP outpaces the ability to replenish the supply from circulating creatine phosphate. The anaerobic glycolysis system is prevalent in the initial phases of sporting activity or extremely high-intensity sporting activities, as determined by the percentage of the VO_2 max. The benefit of this is the athlete gets fast access to energy, but there are a couple of drawbacks. First, the result of anaerobic glycolysis is both the production of energy and lactic acid. Unfortunately, lactic acid will build up during sustained exercise in which the intensity is higher than the body's ability to utilize oxygen. This build-up of lactic acid could lead to muscle fatigue. The second drawback to anaerobic glycolysis as an energy source for more sustained activity is the inability to enter the tricarboxylic acid cycle (TCA) or Krebs cycle due to the lack of oxygen, or more accurately, the requirement for oxygen is higher than the availability. This pathway is most used either while initiating a longer, lower-intensity activity before moving to another energy system or as a primary energy system for high-intensity activity lasting from two to three minutes maximum [4, 5]. Therefore, we can think of many sprinting events and high-intensity sports that fit these constraints events; for example, anaerobic glycolysis is a good fuel source for an 800-m sprint or one shift in hockey but would not be suitable for an entire hockey game or practice unless the player had enough rest between shifts. Recovery from the anaerobic glycolytic system is based on the removal of lactic acid. A recovery of 95% is expected, or more accurately, the removal of lactic acid can be seen around 30 minutes after finishing an activity. As mentioned, this energy system is ideally used as a way station before a more sustainable energy system takes over or is used during short-duration, high-intensity activities.

2.5.4 Aerobic Glycolysis

Aerobic glycolysis is the energy system that is most commonly thought of with athletic events. This is the energy system that will come into play for activities whose duration is longer than three minutes and whose intensity is lower. In this pathway, after going through both the phosphagen system and anaerobic glycolysis reactions first. We are left with pyruvic acid as the result of glycolysis, which is then able to enter the tricarboxylic acid cycle, otherwise known as the Krebs cycle. Beta-oxidation can be used if fatty acids are going to be the primary fuel source before entering the tricarboxylic acid cycle for the production of ATP. Less commonly, protein can be used as a fuel source as well. The Krebs cycle allows the athletes to generate far more ATP due to the presence of oxygen. The required presence of oxygen makes the VO_2 max an important determinant factor. In other words, if we move the athlete past the 85% VO_2 max load, we enter an oxygen threshold where the oxygen requirement to continue the TCA cycle exceeds the replenishment rate of oxygen, and more lactic acid is built up into the system. It is for this reason that this energy system is utilized for activities that last longer in duration and are lower in overall intensity.

2.5.5 Intensity

In discussing the energy systems used to fuel the athlete during training or competition, the intensity of the sport and phase of training play an important factor to be considered. Not only does the intensity of the activity inform the nutritional professional about the energy system being used but also provides important information about the predominant fuel source for that energy system. The phosphagen system, for example, is going to rely on circulating ATP and creatine phosphate. The conversion process there is relatively straightforward. Anaerobic glycolysis is used during the first two to three minutes and in higher-intensity activities. This energy system will rely on carbohydrates as the primary fuel source. Aerobic glycolysis, on the other hand, will use a combination of fat and carbohydrates for fuel, with a slight preference toward carbohydrates in higher exercise intensities. In exercises with an intensity of greater than 65% of the VO_2 max, we see a shift from fat to carbohydrate as the primary fuel source. The higher the intensity of activity, the more carbohydrates will be used to fuel the activities. Aerobic glycolysis will utilize a higher percentage of fat as the primary fuel source in activities with an intensity of less than 65% of the VO_2 max. Although there will be preferences for which fuel is used primarily based on the intensity of the activity, in most cases, a mixture of carbohydrates and fat will be used to fuel performance [6–10]. It has previously been mentioned that protein can be used as a fuel source for longer durations. Unfortunately, this protein is an inefficient fuel source, which can hurt performance. Additionally, the source of protein can come from diet but also from the breakdown of muscle tissue and should be avoided at all costs. For this reason, we must consider the use of peri-workout nutrition to supply the appropriate amounts of carbohydrates and fats to fuel performance and prevent the use of protein as an energy source for athletes during the performance of training and competition.

One important point that should be made at this point is that although one energy system may be dominant at any given time or level of intensity, more than one energy system can be used by the same sport for different scenarios and phases of training [6]. Let us look at the example of golf. Golf will be practiced as a series of short bursts of activity and then a recovery period. A player takes a shot and either walks or travels via cart to where the ball lands before taking another shot. There is plenty of time in the sport of golf for recovery. Therefore, a golf participant will derive the majority of their energy from the phosphagen system and only a small amount from anaerobic glycolysis. This of course can change as the length of the course increases and the speed at which the athlete will have to complete the course, due to competition or pace of play for other players [11]. On the other hand, a distance runner will go through all three systems, but spend the vast majority of their time in the aerobic glycolytic pathway.

Another factor that also needs to be taken into account when looking at which energy system is dominant used if the athlete is engaged in training vs a competition. This distinction will impact both the intensity and duration of the demands put on the athlete. For example, while a hockey player will spend most of their time in the phosphagen and anaerobic glycolysis zone for a single shift. If we look at the rest periods and the number of shifts involved in the course of the entire game, one expects that hockey player to also use the aerobic glycolysis pathway, as their heart rate will likely be elevated much longer over the course of an entire game. The overall mix will slightly skew heavily toward the phosphagen and anaerobic glycolytic systems. On the other hand, if we look at that same hockey player in practice. We might see an elevated heart rate over the course of a full hour, or longer, but not elevated to the same intensity on average, as a shift in a game. Therefore, a hockey player in practice might utilize a higher percentage of the aerobic glycolysis pathway compared to a hockey player in a game. Another example could include a distance runner who is doing fast-paced work, for example, sprints, at a higher level of intensity during their training, far ahead of the intensity they would be using for a longer distance run. This runner will be using differing mixes of energy systems during training and events which should be accounted for in determining dietary plans [7]. While it may seem pedantic to get into as much detail about energy systems used in different sports and phases of training, it is important that we take into account the demands placed on the body and the specific nutritive requirements of different types of training, competitions, and even the phase of training the athlete may be in. For example, an off-season athlete may use a much higher training volume than an in-season competition training phase, and therefore, their nutritional needs should change. This actually becomes particularly important in weight-dependent sports where we will periodically need to reduce the total caloric intake for the athlete while providing the appropriate macronutrient distribution to fuel the required athletic activities.

2.5.6 Case Study – Jim

Jim is a 37-year-old who competes in an adult hockey league. He has practiced with his team one night a week and games two nights a week. On an additional night, if there is time, he works with a coach on skating speed, edgework, and shooting. This skill-based work is slower-paced with a lot of instruction and fewer repetitions. The weekly practice is one hour long and involves conditioning and team-based play, this consists of a lot of repetitions with medium levels of rest between repetitions. His games often have a higher-than-normal activity level due to the poor attendance of his teammates. Often Steve feels as if he is on the ice every other shift. The game itself is fast paced maximal exertions for 1–1.5 minutes with rest periods of 1–1.5 minutes on average. Given this information alone:

Question:

What energy systems would be dominant during the different activities and how does this impact nutritional recommendations?

Answer:

Steve's skill-based practices involve a lot of rest and fewer repetitions, so this practice is likely going to be more phosphagen system dominant.

The weekly practice is more intensive overall but still has more rest period. While over the course of the hour, Steve will likely be using aerobic glycolysis, the majority of the time will utilize the anaerobic glycolytic system with an emphasis on carbohydrates during the short burst activities. The two games are at a much higher intensity with minimal rest, making it a longer sustained aerobic activity with periodic high-intensity bursts. Due to the fact that he is spending almost half of this time with a higher intensity, he will be using the aerobic glycolytic system predominately with a higher percentage of nutrients being from carbohydrate sources.

2.6 Conclusion

Although an in-depth study of the biochemistry of nutrition and exercise science is beyond the scope of this book, it is no less important that the nutritional consultant or coach be familiar with these principles to better assist their athletes. Collaborating with athletes involves an understanding of the energy systems involved in their sport and how this impacts their nutritive needs to fuel performance and recovery. This is a key consideration when developing a customized dietary protocol for an athlete. An understanding of the basic principles of biochemistry and how the athlete will generate energy from the nutrients they consume will allow for the nutritional provider or coach to better assist the athlete in attaining their goals.

References

1 Gropper SS, Smith JL. *Advanced Nutrition and Human Metabolism*. Cengage Learning, 2018.
2 Ament W, Verkerke GJ. Exercise and fatigue. *Sports Med.* 2009;39(5):389–422. doi:10.2165/00007256-200939050-00005. PMID: 19402743
3 Brooks GA, Mercier J. Balance of carbohydrate and lipid utilization during exercise: the "crossover" concept. *J. Appl. Physiol. (1985)*. 1994;76(6):2253–2261. doi:10.1152/jappl.1994.76.6.2253. PMID: 7928844
4 Sahlin K. Muscle energetics during explosive activities and potential effects of nutrition and training. *Sports Med.* 2014;44(Suppl 2):S167–S173. doi:10.1007/s40279-014-0256-9
5 Melkonian EA, Schury MP. *Biochemistry, Anaerobic Glycolysis*. [Updated 2023 Jul 31]. In: StatPearls [Internet]. Treasure Island (FL): StatPearls Publishing, 2024. Available from: https://www.ncbi.nlm.nih.gov/books/NBK546695/

6 Gastin PB. Energy system interaction and relative contribution during maximal exercise. *Sports Med.* 2001;31(10):725–741. doi:10.2165/00007256-200131100-00003

7 Robergs RA, Ghiasvand F, Parker D. Biochemistry of exercise-induced metabolic acidosis. *Am. J. Physiol. Regul. Integr. Comp. Physiol.* 2004;287(3):R502–R516. doi:10.1152/ajpregu.00114.2004

8 van Loon LJ, Greenhaff PL, Constantin-Teodosiu D, Saris WH, Wagenmakers AJ. The effects of increasing exercise intensity on muscle fuel utilisation in humans. *J. Physiol.* 2001;536(Pt 1):295–304. doi:10.1111/j.1469-7793.2001.00295.x

9 De Feo P, Di Loreto C, Lucidi P, et al. Metabolic response to exercise. *J. Endocrinol. Invest.* 2003;26(9):851–854. doi:10.1007/BF03345235

10 Turcotte LP. Role of fats in exercise. Types and quality. *Clin. Sports Med.* 1999;18(3):485–498. doi:10.1016/s0278-5919(05)70163-0

11 Zoffer M. Competitive golf: how longer courses are changing athletes and their approach to the game. *Nutrients* 2022;14(9):1732. Published 2022 Apr 22. doi:10.3390/nu14091732

3

The Aging Process

3.1 Introduction

Sports nutrition, as a field of study, has the potential to impact athletic performance both in positive, if applied efficiently, and negative ways, if misapplied. Although sports nutrition has the potential to impact sports performance for all athletes the impact that sports nutrition can have on older athletes is particularly significant given the physiological changes the older athlete will have seen in their life as they age. Many of the changes impacting older athletes come from alterations in the normal physiological processes that occur as part of the overall aging process, such as metabolic slowdown or loss of bone density. Other changes that impact older athletes involve acquired conditions due to medical and lifestyle considerations, such as diabetes or atherosclerosis. These changes are not unique to athletes, but their impact can significantly affect performance. It is essential, therefore, that anyone working with an older athletic population understand the physiological changes that can impact the aging athlete, and by understanding these changes, the nutritional professional will be better equipped to design an appropriate eating strategy. This chapter will focus on the changes in physiology that occur as part of the aging process.

Getting older is a fact of life; the impacts of aging affect everyone but to differing degrees. Unfortunately, the impact of aging hits a little harder when looking at the performance of athletes. The process of aging will impact performance through all age levels, from youth athletes all the way up to masters age group athletes. Youth athletes will see an enhancement in performance as they age and mature. Older athletes, on the other hand, will see a decline in their performance as they age. The physiological effects of aging impact the athlete's ability to recover from exercise and perform optimally in their chosen sport. Changes that the body will experience, and

Sports Nutrition for Masters Athletes, First Edition. Peter G. Nickless.
© 2025 John Wiley & Sons, Inc. Published 2025 by John Wiley & Sons, Inc.

the extent to which the athlete experiences them, should be understood as they will affect the needs of the athlete in terms of training programming, recovery plans, and most importantly for this book, the nutritional plan needed to support the athlete. It would, therefore, make sense that any conversation about aging and the nutritional needs of aging athletes needs to talk about the physiologic and performance-based changes an athlete can expect to see as they get older.

The effects of aging are widespread and include, amongst others, changes in the motor neurons, changes in the endocrine system (specifically changes in hormonal production and balance), and changes in how oxygen is delivered to cells. It is by taking these changes into account and through continued training, nutrition, and planned recovery that we can help ameliorate some of the deficits seen as a result of aging for athletes. Although the point of this book is to focus on the nutritional considerations needed to optimize athletic performance, it is essential to note the impact of continued athletic performance and the role of this performance in maintaining athletic capabilities, meaning the act of training itself can help the athlete to reduce some of the impacts of aging. Through the understanding of the physiologic impacts of aging we will see how nutrition aimed at supporting recovery and performance can be an important training aid to fuel this training as the athlete ages.

3.2 Performance-Based Changes

As all people age, there is an expectation that the normal physiologic aging process will lead to a decline in performance from a peak; this decline in performance will have differing impacts on athletes. They may mean a reduction in 100 m sprint speed for a track and field athletes or simply a quicker time to fatigue for the nonathlete as they perform their activities of daily living, such as walking. Typically, this performance decline will start in the adult's mid to late 30s. It is expected that on average older athletes will not perform physical activities as well as they did when they were younger. The athlete who was quick in their 20s will start to lose a step and slow in their 30s. This does not mean that there cannot be some exceptionally performing older athletes, only that physiologically they are typically not performing as well as they did when they were younger. These changes may not always be as easy to notice as some sports allow the athlete to change their game as they age, letting them to continue to compete despite a changing toolset. A hockey player who was more of an explosive athlete who relied on quick bursts of speed to score may become better at stickhandling and passing, altering their game to that of a more of technical player.

This loss in neuromuscular performance usually accounts for approximately a 2–4% decline in strength and power per year [1]. While it would be nice to be able to predict the rate of decline an athlete will experience, it is typically nonlinear. Performance decline cannot be mapped out directly or predicted accurately, but this average decline will be seen over a period of time. Overall, there would be evidence that a nontrained individual could lose much of their strength annually as they pass the age of 35. Assuming the individual has not been working out consistently and we are just assessing pure untrained strength. It is therefore not unreasonable to think that an individual in their 70s could see over a 50% decrease in their leg strength. These changes can be significant when we take into account the impact that a 50% strength decline can have on things like activities of daily living. Take, for example, getting up from a seated position, or from a fall, if the individual has trouble getting up from the floor at age 40 imagine the impact that three to four decades of performance decline can have. The changes can have a profound impact on the individual's quality and potential quantity of life. It is important to note that this change specifically mentioned the decreased performance in individuals who do not train. Athletes who maintain a training regime can slow these numbers significantly allowing an older athlete to maintain much of their 35-year-old performance capacity. This serves to drive home the fact that although there is going to be a decline in athletic performance seen as one ages, these changes are not absolute and can be directly linked to and reduced by continued activity [2–5]. This is also a strong argument for continued participation in training and physical activity as one ages. The real-world impact would mean that through proper training and focus on recovery, there can be a reduction in the rate at which an athlete will experience a decline in their performance and through training to minimize some of the physiologic impacts of aging on performance. This would serve to not only provide inspiration to athletes, but frankly all individuals, to follow a training regime as they age. Although the focus on this book is to focus on the nutritional needs of older athletes to maintain this level of performance, it is important to note the need for a well-designed exercise plan to help the athlete maintain as high a level of performance that they are capable of for as long as possible.

3.3 Motor Neuron Changes

In the nervous system, nerve cells are separated into different types of cells based on functionality such as motor and sensory neurons. A motor neuron is a nerve cell connecting from the central nervous system to muscle fibers. The motor neuron and the associated muscle cells they connect to are called a motor unit. This serves as the connection point between the nervous and muscular systems. Motor neurons, among other things, transmit impulses from the brain to signal the muscles that it is time for a contraction. This connection between the nervous and muscular systems is essential not only to initiate muscle contraction but also to control the amplitude of the muscular contraction. In short, without motor neurons and motor units, there can be no voluntary muscle contractions. Motor units are associated with both Type 1 (AKA fast twitch) muscle fibers and Type 2 (AKA slow twitch) muscle fibers. Fast twitch muscle fibers are associated with explosive contractions but are quick to fatigue, whereas slow twitch fibers do not fatigue as quickly but also will contract slower. Accordingly, it is through the use of motor neurons that we can regulate muscle contraction speed and force. It would, therefore, be essential to maintain our functioning motor units as long as possible. A sedentary or inactive adult can see as much as a 30–40% motor unit loss compared to younger athletes. This will lead to decreased muscle mass and a potential decrease in athletic performance through losses in muscular strength and endurance. Decreased motor neurons are associated with sarcopenia, which is the loss of muscle mass, and dynapenia, which is the loss of muscular strength due to aging. Active adults will see less decline in motor neurons and as a result have the potential to maintain a greater functional capacity for muscular contraction over a longer time [1, 3–5]. This effect of training and proper nutrition to fuel and recover from training may be important for both maintaining performance and healthy movement as the athlete ages.

3.4 Endocrine Changes

The endocrine system is made up of the glands and hormones that help to control homeostatic balance in the body. It is through the endocrine system that the body can control mechanisms such as growth and metabolism. These functions are accomplished through proper balance of hormones such as growth hormone, testosterone, calcitonin, and insulin among others. The functions of the endocrine system carry particular importance as they relate to athletic performance and the recovery of an athlete from training and competition. The aging process can bring on various changes to how the endocrine system functions, specifically in relation to changes in hormonal production, and balance. Typically, these changes are associated with reductions in the secretion of hormones. Endocrine changes will impact a variety of bodily functions, specifically the hormones that are associated with recovery and performance. It is through a well-designed training program combined with appropriately planned nutritional interventions aimed at reducing the effects of some of these endocrine changes that we can help the athlete to a greater effect on maintaining or improving performance as the athlete ages. Let us examine some of the hormonal changes associated with the aging processes.

Growth hormone or somatotrophin is a hormone produced by the pituitary gland that is responsible for the growth, development, and repair of tissues. The production and secretion of growth hormone will peak during adolescence and decrease as the individual ages. The decline in growth hormone will negatively impact muscle recovery, muscle fiber number, size, and strength. There are also other negative changes associated with the loss of growth hormone such as the increase in body fat deposition, and loss of bone density. These will have a negative impact on both athletic performance and general health. Considering the expected decline in growth hormone over time it is also reasonable to assume the decline in growth hormone has a negative impact on athletic performance. There is an ongoing debate as to the potential negative health impact of synthetic growth hormone administration. There is some evidence to support the use of growth hormone for athletic improvement and performance due to its role in increasing muscle mass, improving recovery, and decreasing body fat. On the other hand, there is evidence linking elevations in growth hormone with decreases in health and longevity particularly seen with conditions associated with the cardiovascular system and insulin sensitivity. This would indicate that although growth hormone plays a role in sports performance there must be a control of growth hormone within a distinct range where we can see maximal performance benefit without negatively impacting longevity. Additionally, synthetic growth hormone is only available by prescription and is, with limited exception, a banned substance for athletes competing in drug-tested sporting events. It would therefore be ideal to target strategies to maximize the internal production of growth hormone. Nutritional and lifestyle changes may have some impact on reducing the impact of growth hormone reduction and loss. Strenuous exercise, stress reduction, and sleep, for example, are lifestyle changes that can increase internal growth hormone production. Keep in mind that strenuous exercise must be accompanied by a recovery period for full effect. Nutritionally reducing sugar consumption, increasing protein consumption, intermittent fasting, and supplements such as arginine, GABA, and citrulline have been shown to increase growth hormone secretion, although there is some debate regarding the effect of supplementing amino acids on athletes [6–9].

Vasopressin is a hormone that has vital functions related to fluid balance and kidney function, and by extension helps to control blood pressure.

Another term for vasopressin is anti-diuretic hormone. As the name suggests, the role of this hormone is to reduce diuresis or the loss of water from the system by increasing water reuptake in the kidneys. Increases in vasopressin would decrease urination, whereas decreases in vasopressin will lead to increased urination. In either extreme, for deviations from the normal range, there is a potential negative outcome. Let us use the example of decreased vasopressin: alcohol consumption decreases vasopressin, which leads to increases in urination and can lead to the symptoms of dehydration and has a role in the feelings associated with a hangover. Secretion of vasopressin fluctuates during the day; as an individual ages, there is often a disruption in the normal cycling of vasopressin; there is also a reduction in the thirst mechanism. The suppression of this hormone is more likely to lead to excess urination and fluid loss, while the decreased thirst mechanism can lead to a state of negative fluid balance [6, 10]. The impact of this will make the athlete more prone to dehydration and concomitant performance loss. Performance strategies need to focus on maintaining fluid balance so that the athlete will not be at an increased risk of dehydration and performance loss. As the athlete ages there is a greater import placed on strategies to prevent dehydration. Chapter 7 will go into hydration strategies in more detail.

Melatonin is a hormone produced by the pineal gland. Synthesized from the metabolism of the amino acid tryptophan, melatonin is associated with circadian rhythms regulating the sleep–wake cycle. Melatonin production peaks in young children and declines significantly until the individual reaches adulthood. Melatonin production is further diminished in individuals as they age. The effects of decreased melatonin on sleep–wake cycles can have health-related changes, such as an increased risk for cardiovascular disease, obesity, and diseases related to obesity. This decline will have a particular impact on athletes as decreased melatonin can be seen with increases in recovery times and regeneration from post-exercise sleep loss. The restorative impacts of sleep are an important part of recovery for athletes, and a reduction in sleep is directly associated with reduced performance. Interventions can be aimed at maximizing potential melatonin production, through lifestyle modifications or through direct supplementation of melatonin [6, 11]. The goal of increasing melatonin in athletes is aimed at increasing the amount of restful sleep enabling how the athlete is able to recover fully from exercise. Other benefits of increased melatonin include the reduction in oxidative stress and improvements in the control of inflammation. Older athletes should consider melatonin supplementation as part of their overall training plan.

Cortisol is a hormone produced by the adrenal glands. This hormone is often considered by athletes to be a negative one, but in reality, it has quite a few important functions for helping to maintain homeostatic balance. Cortisol is associated with the typical stress response, it is associated with the reduction of inflammation, blood pressure regulation, protein and fat metabolism, and glucose control and regulation. Cortisol must be kept within a specific range; too little cortisol can interfere with normal physiologic functions, but too much can also lead to a disruption in these functions. Cortisol is a catabolic hormone and, in excess, can have a negative impact on hormone production, sleep regulation, weight gain, muscle repair, and tissue regeneration. The production of cortisol declines as we age, although older athletes must be careful, as exercising beyond their capacity to recover will elevate cortisol levels. As described, both low and high cortisol levels can lead to issues that will negatively impact the athlete's performance and, accordingly, must be kept to a specific range. Nutritional and lifestyle modifications can have an impact on hormone production to assist the athlete in maintaining appropriate cortisol levels. Lifestyle modifications to reduce the negative impacts of cortisol involve increase sleep, meditation, light exercise, avoiding caffeine, and stress avoidance. Nutritionally, cortisol levels can be reduced through diet dietary changes including high in healthy fats, high in antioxidants, and probiotics. Some supplements aimed at reducing cortisol include but are not limited to ashwagandha, phosphatidylserine, theanine, and magnesium [12, 13].

The hormones epinephrine and norepinephrine, produced by the adrenal glands, help to mediate the stress response. These two hormones are involved in the "fight or flight" sympathetic nervous system reactions. While epinephrine has its actions on the heart rate, blood sugar control, and lung expansion, norepinephrine has its impact on blood vessels, through constriction, which leads to increased blood pressure and flow. These hormones work together to provide increased blood flow to tissues, bringing oxygen and nutrients, in order to respond to stressors. The role of epinephrine and norepinephrine can be seen in athletes as they use this increased blood flow for training and competition. These two hormones see a reduction in secretion for older individuals, which can impair athletic performance through decreased action. Although less in quantity, the hormones often stay in circulation longer, possibly mitigating some of the impact of their reduction. Overtraining, which is more common in older athletes, can lead to elevations in epinephrine, norepinephrine, and cortisol, which can lead to a catabolic breakdown in muscle tissue and decreased athletic performance [13–15]. A well-designed training plan is essential to reduce epinephrine and norepinephrine.

Thyroid hormones T3 and T4 are produced in the thyroid and controlled by the hormone thyroid-stimulating hormone produced by the anterior pituitary gland. These hormones are important in controlling metabolism and energy production, the metabolism of the macronutrients carbohydrates, fats, and proteins, and for protein synthesis. It is through these roles that the thyroid hormones will have an impact on athletic performance. Thyroid hormone production will decline as a normal part of the aging process. However, the response of the thyroid hormone can be different and individual. Some may see an increase in production, while some may see a decline. The impact of low thyroid hormone can be similar to aging, with symptoms like fatigue, low pulse, poor cold temperature tolerance, difficulty breathing, and slowed recovery. There are various reasons for this, from an age-related primary decline to a secondary reaction to an underlying health condition. Excess thyroid production can lead to heat intolerance, anxiety, sweating, tremors, difficulty sleeping, and undesired weight loss. All of which can negatively impact the athlete's performance. It is essential that thyroid function be assessed and monitored by a medical professional, as a medical intervention may be required. Nutrition may have an impact on thyroid hormone production and should be addressed as well. Nutritional considerations include foods containing iodine and selenium [16–18].

Testosterone and estrogen are the sex hormones produced in the testicles and the ovaries, respectively. Testosterone is responsible for the maturation and development in males and is associated with muscle mass and strength in both males and females. Estrogen is responsible for secondary sex characteristics in females. Estrogen is more associated with decreased performance in males, if levels are too high. Both testosterone and estrogen are made by both males and females, although to differing degrees. As the athlete ages, there is a decline in testosterone production, which can negatively impact performance. In females, estrogen levels will decrease, which can increase the risk of bone fractures, while in males, levels of estrogen will increase, which can lead to decreased muscle mass and performance. Supplemental testosterone is banned for male athletes; estrogen can be used for female athletes with a medical waiver. Nutrition strategies should be focused on maintaining stable production of testosterone and estrogen [19, 20].

3.5 Oxygen Delivery Changes

As people age, there is a decrease in the body's ability to deliver oxygen to tissues. Some of this has been addressed in the changes listed earlier. In addition to the aforementioned changes, age will bring on a decline in the maximal heart rate. Maximum heart rate can be calculated by 220 minus your age. This decrease in the maximal heart rate will decrease the body's ability to deliver oxygen to tissues to generate muscle performance. There is also a decline in the number of mitochondria, which is the primary source of ATP production. This will decrease the body's ability to produce ATP for use as an energy source to fuel activity. Additionally, there is a decrease in the VO_2 max. The VO_2 max represents the maximum amount of oxygen that can be delivered to the muscles during exercise. Unfortunately, this decrease will have a significant impact on the body's ability to deliver oxygen to working muscles and will result in a decrease in the time to fatigue. This change will have a larger impact on endurance athletes. Training, diet, and lifestyle modifications will help to mitigate some of the impact of oxygen delivery changes. Nutritional strategies should be aimed at increasing or maintaining red blood cell production, maintaining blood vessel health, and improving mitochondria [21, 22].

3.6 Conclusion

The aging process is complex, having effects on all of the 11 organ systems individually, and in many cases, impacting how they interact with each other. For example, losses in muscle mass are going to impact the ability of the nervous system to control fine motor movement. Conversely, losses in motor neuronal function will have impacts on the body's ability to interact with the muscular system to perform complex tasks quickly. These impacts, whether they are large or small, will have effects on the athlete's ability to perform their chosen sport to their best and will impact their athletic goals. In short, the physiological effects of aging bring on changes that will decrease the athlete's performance capabilities. Despite these changes, evidence supports that the use of focused dietary strategies, lifestyle modifications, and a well-designed training plan that includes adequate recovery can help to combat the impacts of aging physiologically, allowing the athlete to perform at a higher level for a longer period of time.

References

1 Lavin KM, Roberts BM, Fry CS, et al. The importance of resistance exercise training to combat neuromuscular aging. *Physiol. (Bethesda)* 2019;34(2):112–122. doi:10.1152/physiol.00044.2018
2 Norheim KL, Hjort Bønløkke J, Samani A, Omland Ø, Madeleine P. The effect of aging on physical performance among elderly manual workers: protocol of a cross-sectional study. *JMIR Res. Protoc.* 2017;6(11):e226. Published 2017 Nov 22. doi:10.2196/resprot.8196

3 Tanaka H, Tarumi T, Rittweger J. Aging and physiological lessons from master athletes. *Compr. Physiol.* 2019;10(1):261-296. Published 2019 Dec 18. doi:10.1002/cphy.c180041

4 American College of Sports Medicine Position Stand. Exercise and physical activity for older adults. *Med. Sci. Sports Exerc.* 1998;30(6):992-1008.

5 Hunter GR, McCarthy JP, Bamman MM. Effects of resistance training on older adults. *Sports Med.* 2004;34(5):329-348. doi:10.2165/00007256-200434050-00005

6 van den Beld AW, Kaufman JM, Zillikens MC, et al. The physiology of endocrine systems with ageing. *Lancet Diabetes Endocrinol.* 2018;6(8):647-658. doi:10.1016/S2213-8587(18)30026-3

7 Hage C, Salvatori R. Growth hormone and aging. *Endocrinol. Metab. Clin. North Am.* 2023;52(2):245-257. doi:10.1016/j.ecl.2022.10.003

8 Cummings DE, Merriam GR. Age-related changes in growth hormone secretion: should the somatopause be treated?*Semin. Reprod. Endocrinol.* 1999;17(4):311-325. doi:10.1055/s-2007-1016241

9 Caputo M, Pigni S, Agosti E, et al. Regulation of GH and GH signaling by nutrients. *Cells* 2021;10(6):1376. Published 2021 Jun 2. doi:10.3390/cells10061376

10 Duffy JF, Scheuermaier K, Loughlin KR. Age-related sleep disruption and reduction in the circadian rhythm of urine output: contribution to nocturia?*Curr. Aging Sci.* 2016;9(1):34-43. doi:10.2174/1874609809666151130220343

11 Verma AK, Khan MI, Ashfaq F, Rizvi SI. Crosstalk between aging, circadian rhythm, and melatonin. *Rejuvenation Res.* 2023;26(6):229-241. doi:10.1089/rej.2023.0047

12 Stamou MI, Colling C, Dichtel LE. Adrenal aging and its effects on the stress response and immunosenescence. *Maturitas.* 2023;168:13-19. doi:10.1016/j.maturitas.2022.10.006

13 Hill EE, Zack E, Battaglini C, et al. Exercise and circulating cortisol levels: the intensity threshold effect. *J. Endocrinol. Invest.* 2008;31(7):587-591. doi:10.1007/BF03345606

14 Esler M, Kaye D, Thompson J, et al. Effects of aging on epinephrine secretion and regional release of epinephrine from the human heart. *J. Clin. Endocrinol. Metab.* 1995;80(2):435-442. doi:10.1210/jcem.80.2.7852502

15 Yiallouris A, Tsioutis C, Agapidaki E, et al. Adrenal aging and its implications on stress responsiveness in humans. *Front. Endocrinol. (Lausanne)* 2019;10:54. Published 2019 Feb 7. doi:10.3389/fendo.2019.00054

16 Leng O, Razvi S. Hypothyroidism in the older population. *Thyroid Res.* 2019;12:2. Published 2019 Feb 8. doi:10.1186/s13044-019-0063-3

17 Gesing A, Lewiński A, Karbownik-Lewińska M. The thyroid gland and the process of aging; what is new? *Thyroid Res.* 2012;5(1):16. Published 2012 Nov 24. doi:10.1186/1756-6614-5-16
18 Duhig TJ, McKeag D. Thyroid disorders in athletes. *Curr. Sports Med. Rep.* 2009;8(1):16–19. doi:10.1249/JSR.0b013e3181954a12
19 Ketchem JM, Bowman EJ, Isales CM. Male sex hormones, aging, and inflammation. *Biogerontology* 2023;24(1):1–25. doi:10.1007/s10522-022-10002-1
20 Horstman AM, Dillon EL, Urban RJ, Sheffield-Moore M. The role of androgens and estrogens on healthy aging and longevity. *J. Gerontol. A Biol. Sci. Med. Sci.* 2012;67(11):1140–1152. doi:10.1093/gerona/gls068
21 Marzetti E, Calvani R, Coelho-Júnior HJ, Landi F, Picca A. Mitochondrial quantity and quality in age-related sarcopenia. *Int. J. Mol. Sci.* 2024;25(4):2052. Published 2024 Feb 8. doi:10.3390/ijms25042052
22 Guo Y, Guan T, Shafiq K, et al. Mitochondrial dysfunction in aging. *Ageing Res. Rev.* 2023;88:101955. doi:10.1016/j.arr.2023.101955

4

Macronutrients

4.1 Introduction

All people, athletes and nonathletes alike, require energy to carry on the activities of daily life. Energy is needed to support these essential functions such as cellular processes, metabolism, and respiration as well as nonvital functions such as movement and exercise. Athletic performance requires adequate energy to perform any exercise at all, let alone at optimal levels. This energy comes in the form of adenosine triphosphate (ATP). In breaking the bonds that hold the phosphate groups to ATP, breaking ATP to ADP, energy is released. Energy is required to fuel the cells involved in athletic performance. This energy need is met through consuming and metabolizing macronutrients. Making macronutrients essential for both homeostatic balance and athletic performance. The term macronutrient is used to classify nutrients that can be metabolized to provide the body with the substrate needed to satisfy energy requirements and carry on the physiological processes necessary for survival. Athletes use these macronutrients to meet their energy needs to support the recovery and fueling requirements to participate in sports. The three macronutrients, carbohydrates, proteins, and fats (or lipids) are required in larger quantities and must be supplied by the diet to meet these requirements. The human body cannot produce these nutrients on its own, making them essential to be provided from the diet; the only exception to this are carbohydrates, which are not essential as they can be created through alternative biochemical processes, such as gluconeogenesis. The energy produced from macronutrients comes in the form of calories. In the case of food, the stored energy is found within the cellular structure of the food. This potential energy is converted to kinetic energy

Sports Nutrition for Masters Athletes, First Edition. Peter G. Nickless.
© 2025 John Wiley & Sons, Inc. Published 2025 by John Wiley & Sons, Inc.

through a series of biochemical metabolic processes to be discussed in this chapter. While some energy is used in these biochemical processes, these processes signify the transformation of food to more usable energy sources for cellular function, growth, and repair. The macronutrients are broken down into their simplest forms for absorption and utilization. Carbohydrates are absorbed as monosaccharides, proteins as amino acids, and lipids as fatty acids. We will discuss these more in subsequent sections.

4.2 Carbohydrates

Carbohydrates carry out several functions in the body. Among these, energy production is the most important. Although alternative means of creating energy exist, carbohydrates are the diet's primary energy source. Carbohydrates can provide an instant form of energy for immediate use, a stored form of energy in the form of glycogen for later use, and a steady form of energy through biochemical pathways. Carbohydrates are necessary for optimal athletic performance and have a role in fueling both the performance and recovery of athletes from training and competition.

4.2.1 Carbohydrates and Intensity

Dietary carbohydrates are important and the most prominent energy source athletes use for their activity. The extent to which carbohydrates play a role in exercise is related to the intensity of the exercise, although carbohydrates will always play at least some role. Higher-intensity activities will utilize carbohydrates as the primary fuel for activities. Although low- and moderate-intensity activities will use a significant source of fat as their energy source, carbohydrates are still needed to burn fat for energy. As stated, the higher the intensity, the more significant the role of carbohydrates is. In Chapter 2, energy systems and their role in athletic activity were discussed in more detail. Still, the relationship between exercise intensity and carbohydrate use is directly proportional, meaning that as the intensity of the activity increases, the need for carbohydrates will increase [1]. Circulating ATP and stored carbohydrates as glycogen will be the primary fuel source for anaerobic activities. These are exercise activities with high enough intensity where the body cannot get enough oxygen to replenish energy sources. As the exercise intensity decreases and the body can use oxygen to replenish energy stores, a mixture of fuel sources comes in. This is because all other biochemical pathways for energy production are oxygen-dependent.

4.2.2 Carbohydrate Structure and Metabolism

Chemically, carbohydrates contain carbon as the base of their structure, attached to oxygen and hydrogen. Carbohydrates can have one single carbon unit or can be bound to chains that have two or more carbons. Carbohydrates are often classified as simple or complex carbohydrates. Simple carbohydrates include monosaccharides and disaccharides, and complex carbohydrates contain oligosaccharides and polysaccharides.

A monosaccharide, sometimes called a simple sugar, is the simplest type of carbohydrate consisting of only one single carbon molecule. This monosaccharide is the simplest form and is the state in which carbohydrates are digested and metabolized. All carbohydrates are broken into their monosaccharide form for digestion. The three monosaccharides are glucose, fructose, and galactose. In foods, carbohydrates are not commonly seen as monosaccharides by themselves. One good example of a monosaccharide in the diet is the fructose found in fruits. Monosaccharides can also be purchased in supplement forms, for example, glucose tablets. Most simple carbohydrates in the diet that occur naturally in food come from disaccharides, not monosaccharides [2].

Disaccharides are carbohydrate chains that contain two carbon units and are the second simplest form of saccharides. Disaccharides are also classified as simple carbohydrates or simple sugars, along with monosaccharides. Disaccharides found in the diet are sucrose, lactose, and maltose. Disaccharides are made of two combined monosaccharides and broken down into their two monosaccharide components for absorption and metabolism. Sucrose, sometimes called table sugar, can be broken down into one glucose and one fructose molecule for absorption and metabolism. Lactose contains one glucose and one galactose monosaccharide joined together, and maltose contains two glucose molecules joined together. Although all three disaccharides share the similarity of containing two monosaccharides joined, they are not metabolized identically. After being broken down into its two glucose components, maltose will enter the biochemical process of glycolysis to be broken down. On the other hand, sucrose contains one glucose which will enter glycolysis directly, but the fructose molecule will undergo a series of chemical changes in the liver before entering glycolysis. These differences in metabolism can alter the effects of the nutrients and, accordingly, their impact on health and performance; maltose can be broken down into glucose and metabolized more quickly and, therefore, can have a more significant effect on blood sugar when compared to sucrose or lactose [2].

Oligosaccharides are saccharides made of carbon chains of 3–10 carbons. Classified as complex carbohydrates, these saccharide chains will be comprised of multiple units of the monosaccharides glucose, fructose, and galactose. While various oligosaccharides can occur, the most common are oligosaccharides containing four carbons called tetra saccharides. Some examples of oligosaccharides include maltotriose, a trisaccharide with three glucose units, and raffinose, a trisaccharide with one galactose, glucose, and a fructose molecule. These oligosaccharides occur in various foods found in the diet. For example, raffinose can be found in legumes, cabbage, broccoli, brussels sprouts, asparagus, whole grains, etc. Oligosaccharides are not digested by human digestive enzymes but are used as fuel for the bacteria in the intestine. These carbohydrates are prebiotic and carry many of the health benefits associated with prebiotic foods, including, among others, enhanced immune function, improved lipid profile, and improved gut health. Additionally, oligosaccharides are associated with lower insulin response when compared to mono and disaccharides and an increased feeling of fullness, which is associated with fiber-rich foods that are oligosaccharide-rich [2]. Those following a low FODMAP diet for health reasons must limit oligosaccharide consumption to avoid increased symptoms [2].

Polysaccharides are saccharides consisting of 11 or more monosaccharides. Polysaccharides must be broken down into smaller saccharide units to be absorbed and metabolized until they eventually become single carbon monosaccharides (the absorption form). The need to break these down from larger chains to monosaccharide form is why polysaccharides are called complex carbohydrates. Polysaccharides include starch, cellulose, or glycogen. Starch is the most common digestible polysaccharide found in plants and can be found in cereal grains, potatoes, legumes, and many vegetables, such as corn. Cellulose is the major component of the cellular walls of plants. Cellulose is resistant to digestion and is a dietary fiber. Cellulose is not an energy source for the body but can be metabolized by the large intestine [2]. Glycogen is the principal storage form of carbohydrates in humans. Glycogen is stored in the liver and the skeletal muscles and can be used to fuel activities when needed. Glycogen can be broken down into glucose through a process called glycogenolysis. Polysaccharides require more work for absorption and metabolism when compared to mono and disaccharides and, therefore, have less impact on elevating blood glucose, thereby providing energy while not carrying as severe negative health impacts of blood glucose volitivity.

Fiber is a unique form of complex carbohydrate. Fibers are long-chain polysaccharides that humans cannot digest for absorption. Because fiber cannot be absorbed, most fiber, except for resistant starches, cannot be utilized by the body to supply energy needs. The role of fiber in the diet has many health-promoting benefits. One health-promoting adequate fiber is the ability of fiber to increase fecal bulk. Fiber attracts water to the intestinal system, which is absorbed and expands, adding size to fecal matter. The larger the bulk in the intestinal system, the more significant the peristaltic actions of smooth muscles and, accordingly, the faster the passage of food through the digestive system, decreasing transit time. So, increasing fecal bulk will decrease the transit time of food through the gastrointestinal system, leading to fewer issues with constipation compared to individuals consuming a low-fiber diet. Fiber can reduce the risk for certain cancers, for example, colon cancer. This may be due to several factors, including the decreased transit time, which more rapidly reduces exposure to cancer-causing agents. Dietary fiber has also been associated with decreased cholesterol and reduced risk for heart disease. Soluble fiber binds to bile acids in the gastrointestinal tract, which prevents their reabsorption, reducing the amount of cholesterol reducing the risk of cardiovascular disease. Additionally, the short-chain fatty acids produced by the gastrointestinal system may inhibit cholesterol production [2]. Diets high in fiber may have a role in weight management. This is due to fiber's ability to absorb water, increasing fecal bulk. The increased fecal bulk makes a person feel full longer and less likely to overeat.

The current acceptable macronutrient distribution range (AMDR) for carbohydrates is 45–65% of the diet [3]. The AMDR is a general guideline for consumption and is nonspecific to individuals, so the actual percentage needed will fluctuate based on the person and the athletic endeavor. In terms of energy supply, carbohydrates contain 4 calories/g. So, if we were to look at a 2000-calorie diet that consisted of 50% carbohydrates, we would see that 1000 calories come from carbohydrates. If we divide 1000 calories by 4 calories/g, this individual will consume 250 g of carbohydrates.

4.2.3 Carbohydrate Deficiency and Performance

An important role of carbohydrates in an athlete's diet is to prevent the breakdown of protein for utilization to meet energy needs. Although protein can be used to meet the energy needs for exercise, protein has other more important functions. Using protein to produce energy would not be ideal for athletic function. Part of the reason for this is that one method the body can use to metabolize protein for energy would be the breakdown of muscle tissue to get the amino acids needed to produce energy. In this way, carbohydrate consumption can help to reduce muscle breakdown to meet energy needs and, therefore, has a muscle-sparing effect. The benefit to the athlete is not an increase in performance but rather no performance lost due to muscle breakdown.

Another role of adequate carbohydrate consumption in the diet is for nervous system function. The optimal function of the nervous system is also dependent on carbohydrate intake. This is because glucose is the primary fuel source for the brain and nervous system. Carbohydrate deficiency can result in the brain and nervous system needing energy through alternative means. Although these alternative means of providing the brain and nervous system with energy exist, they are not an efficient fuel source. Low carbohydrate consumption can negatively impact athletic performance due to impaired nervous system function. At this point, it is worth mentioning that there are circumstances in which an athlete can adapt to a fat-based diet to fuel performance. This is a complex process and, at least in the short term, can negatively impact performance before complete fat adaptation. For these reasons, carbohydrates are still the preferred macronutrient for fueling energy needs and will be the most used nutrient. We will get into low-carbohydrate diets for athletes in another section later in this chapter.

It has been discussed how dietary fiber can positively impact health for all humans, not just athletes. We also discussed how dietary fiber is a long chain of polysaccharides that is indigestible in the human body. Conversely, simple carbohydrates, mono, and disaccharides will also impact health. First and foremost, simple sugars are a quick source of calories. Often, foods containing large amounts of simple carbohydrates contain more calories per ounce when compared to a higher fibrous food. In other words, an ounce of table sugar will have more calories than an ounce of broccoli. This would indicate two things. First, while there is an increase in energy availability for the athlete, sometimes that energy availability will outpace the requirements for this athlete, leading to fat mass accumulation. Additionally, because there is a lack of bulk in these foods, there will be a decrease in the feeling of fullness associated with simple sugars compared to dietary fiber. This can lead to overconsumption if diets contain foods lower in fiber. Another concern for simple carbohydrates is the increased ability for simple carbohydrates to elevate small particle size, low-density lipoprotein, or LDL cholesterol. LDL cholesterol is associated with an increased risk for cardiovascular disease and is pro-inflammatory which, as discussed in Chapter 9, carries significant health concerns [4]. Finally, simple carbohydrates, particularly in beverages and candy consumption, have been associated with increased dental caries and tooth decay [5]. Looking at the foods that commonly contain more significant percentages of simple carbohydrates, we will also tend to see foods with lower overall nutrient density providing fewer micronutrients per gram than other, more complex carbohydrate sources. Comparatively, this would make them a less ideal nutrient source. An additional concern is that many simple carbohydrate-containing foods in the standard American diet will also have higher quantities of dietary fat content associated with them, which can further increase the caloric density and health implications of the foods. So, if an athlete were to maintain a specific caloric intake, consuming a higher percentage of calories from simple carbohydrates would mean replacing other food options that may be more nutrient-dense, providing more benefit to the athlete. Therefore, there is an opportunity cost where simple carbohydrates replacing more calorically dense, complex carbohydrates can lead to a less nutritious diet overall for the athlete, negatively impacting performance. Considering food choice, it stands to reason that choosing a diet where most carbohydrate needs are met by complex carbohydrates, over simple carbohydrates, will benefit overall health and athletic performance. One caveat is that there may be circumstances within intra and post-workout nutrition where simple sugars may be preferred. Still, these circumstances are targeted explicitly toward peri-workout nutrition and not for general health.

The role of insulin and carbohydrate consumption is an important consideration, as insulin is one of two hormones responsible for regulating blood sugar, the other being glucagon. Insulin is released in response to elevations in blood sugar and works by removing excess sugar in the blood for storage in the liver and muscles as glycogen. Glucagon, on the other hand, is released when blood sugar is too low and functions to increase blood sugar by helping to release stored glycogen from the liver and muscles. As mentioned, insulin responds to elevations in blood sugar; therefore, every carbohydrate consumed will have some impact on blood sugar and insulin. This impact is significant because blood sugar must be maintained within specific parameters. Excess blood sugar stimulates a release of insulin which will lead to the removal of extra sugar from the blood to be stored in the liver or muscles as glycogen through a process called glycogenesis. Conversely, if blood sugar is too low, glucagon is a hormone that increases blood sugar by releasing and breaking down glycogen from the muscle and liver through the process of glycogenolysis. As blood sugar must be maintained within a narrow window, examining the effects of dietary carbohydrates on elevations in blood glucose is crucial. One way to examine the effects of dietary carbohydrates on blood sugar is to use something called the glycemic index.

4.2.4 The Glycemic Index

The glycemic index refers to the elevation in blood sugar resulting from ingesting dietary carbohydrates. The elevations in blood sugar from a consumed carbohydrate are compared to elevations seen with pure glucose, which has a glycemic index of 100. The higher the glycemic index of a food, the more substantial the elevation in blood sugar (see Figure 4.1). The lower the food's glycemic index, the lower the impact on blood sugar. It is important to note that all carbohydrates will impact blood sugar, but not to the same degree. For example, if glucose, the reference carbohydrate, is 100, sucrose, which contains one glucose molecule and one fructose molecule, has a glycemic index of 65. This would indicate that adding the fructose molecule and the increased work of breaking a disaccharide from two carbons to one for absorption and metabolism will lower the glycemic index and reduce the impact on blood sugar. Traditionally, the more complex the carbohydrate is, the lower the glycemic index and the lower the effect on blood sugar. Despite this rule of thumb, evaluating each carbohydrate's impact is still a good practice. The glycemic index is an important tool in assessing dietary carbohydrates and their potential effect on blood sugar. Another consideration beyond simply glycemic index is also the glycemic load of food. The glycemic load is a measurement of blood sugar that considers the impact of a serving size of a food on blood sugar. This distinction is important because it considers the impact of the food as it is consumed. A food with a glycemic load of 10 or less is considered low. A measurement of 11–19 is considered medium, and 20 or higher is regarded as a high glycemic load. A typical example of the difference between glycemic index and glycemic load can be seen with watermelon. Watermelon has a high glycemic index of 72, indicating that it has a higher impact on blood sugar than pure sucrose, AKA table sugar. Some examples of the differences between glycemic index and glycemic load can be seen in Figure 4.1. This would suggest that it could be a poor choice to be included in a diet trying to control or limit blood sugar increases. Still, because watermelon contains so much water, an actual portion of watermelon contains fewer carbohydrates

Food type	Glycemic index	Glycemic load
White bread	71	11
Jasmine rice	106	48
Brown rice	48	22
Dark chocolate	23	6
Milk chocolate	45	11
Instant mashed potato	88	18
English muffin	77	12
Orange	45	7
Strawberries	40	6
Spaghetti	45	18

Figure 4.1 The glycemic index and glycemic load of various foods.

per serving. Therefore, its glycemic load is only 5, indicating less of a real risk of blood sugar elevations. When trying to control blood sugar as an athlete, it is important to consider the impact of food choices on both glycemic index and glycemic load. There may be circumstances where foods with high glycemic indexes or loads may be preferable. Still, these are mostly related to peri-workout nutrition and assume the athlete does not have issues with blood sugar regulation.

4.2.5 Determining Carbohydrate Need

Determining the amount of carbohydrates needed for an athlete depends on the sport being practiced or contested. Different sporting types, intensities, and the duration of the activity will have different requirements for the athlete. Carbohydrates are also required for the metabolism of fat and protein sparing, assuming we are not talking about a fat-adapted athlete. Carbohydrates serve as an important energy source for sports of differing intensities. High-intensity training at 85% or higher of the VO_2 max will utilize carbohydrates as the primary energy source to fuel activity. In contrast, low-intensity exercise will require carbohydrates, even if it is not the only energy source. Both high- and low-intensity exercises will require carbohydrates but not to the same degree or level. Additionally, as stated when discussing exercise physiology and energy sources, carbohydrates become critical when performing longer-duration exercise to prevent using protein as an energy source. So, the duration of the activity should also be considered for carbohydrate requirements. For example, to complete a 1-hour hockey practice, the athlete may draw on a different mixture of energy sources when compared to a 10-hour mountain climb, but both need to be fueled optimally. The following discuss some of the different carbohydrate recommendations based on the athletic demand of various athletic associations (Figure 4.2). The first example is the American College of Sports Medicine, which recommends that athletes consume between 6 and 10 g of carbohydrates per kilogram of body weight per day. They do not specifically differentiate the type of activity being contested or the intensity of the activity. However, activity intensity can be considered within the ACSM range, with higher-intensity workouts needing closer to 10 g/kg and lower-intensity workouts needing closer to 6 g/kg. The International Society of Sports Nutrition has general physical activity requiring 3–5 g/kg of body weight per day vs high-volume/high-intensity training requiring 8–10 g/kg of body weight per day. The International Olympic Committee uses a carbohydrate requirement range from 3 to 5 g/kg for low-intensity or skill-based activities to high-intensity exercise requiring 8–12 g/kg of body weight per day [6].

Carbohydrate recommendations	
American College of Sports Medicine	
All athletes	6–10 g/kg
International Society of Sports Nutritionists	
General activity	3–5 g/kg
Moderate to high-intensity exercise	5–8 g/kg
High volume exercise	8–10 g/kg
International Olympic Committee	
Low intensity	3–5 g/kg
Moderate intensity	5–7 g/kg
Endurance athletes	6–10 g/kg
Strength athletes	4–7 g/kg
High intensity	8–12 g/kg

Figure 4.2 Recommended requirements for dietary carbohydrates. *Source:* Data from Potgieter [6].

While these charts may demonstrate a wide range of carbohydrate requirements, you will see some continuity between the charts (see Figure 4.2). This could include perspectives about how different the organizations consider the intensity of the contested sports. For example, in all instances, a high-intensity activity will probably need a carbohydrate requirement nearing 10 g/kg of body weight. That amount is relatively consistent for all three organizations. Confusion or difficulty tends to come into play when considering the intensity or volume of training for different sports with subtle differences between them. At the same time, it is more apparent when we look at ultramarathon runners, where the requirements are clearer. When working with strength athletes, there is a need for further clarification regarding intensity and workout duration. It is important to remember the time spent on these activities. For example, 20 minutes at moderate intensity will differ from 2 hours at moderate intensity. This should be considered to determine where we need to place the athlete in the aforementioned carbohydrate recommendation ranges. For example, if the athlete were to go to the gym and lift weights for higher repetitions in the range of 60–70% of their maximum capacity during a one-hour workout. The duration and overall volume likely make this athlete fall into the moderate intensity range, which coincides with 5–7 g/kg, using the International

Olympic Committee Range. Thus, we will discuss this later in the book when we put this information into practice.

4.3 Protein

Protein is an essential macronutrient in the diet. Functionally, protein can be classified as either structural, with muscle tissue as an example, or functional, with enzymes as an example. Proteins are made up of amino acids. For digestion and absorption, proteins are broken down into individual amino acids. Amino acids are the building blocks of protein and carry an important role for the athlete as they provide the raw material necessary to recover from exercise and improve athletic performance. Amino acids can be defined as either essential or nonessential. The body cannot produce essential amino acids, so they must be consumed either as part of the diet or as a supplement. A nonessential amino acid, on the other hand, can be synthesized within the body and does not need to be consumed in large quantities. An important note, however, is that nonessential amino acids can become essential if their requirement for tissue recovery and regeneration exceeds the amount that can be or has been produced within the body. In this case, the amino acid becomes conditionally essential and must be either obtained from the diet or supplementation. A protein containing all essential amino acids is called a complete protein. Since most animal proteins have all essential amino acids, animal proteins are said to be complete. On the other hand, plant proteins are often lacking in one or more essential amino acids and are often incomplete proteins [2]. For this reason, plant protein is often criticized for being of lesser quality than animal protein. It is important to note that proteins of different sources, regardless of completeness, will contain a different mix of amino acids. Incomplete proteins can complement each other and, when combined in sufficient quantities, can create a complete protein or, more accurately, provide the same essential amino acids as a complete protein. An example of combining two incomplete proteins is rice and beans. The protein found in rice and beans is incomplete by itself. Still, in combination, each has the protein missing from the other, providing the amino acid equivalent of a complete protein. In this manner, it is possible for athletes who consume plant-based diets to be able to satisfy their protein needs. The only caveat is that meeting all of the athlete's needs will be more difficult but possible. Conversations about protein quality often refer to the content of essential amino acids they contain (i.e., completeness of the protein), but this is only part of the picture. While a complete protein will have all essential amino acids, completeness alone is not enough to make it the ideal protein to meet the daily requirements of the athlete.

4.3.1 Assessing Protein Quality

We can use several methods to assess protein quality based on type. The most common of these methods is a simple amino acid score. This score represents the percent of the protein's essential amino acids or completeness. This would, of course, be compared to a reference complete protein, usually casein. Since casein is the protein of comparison, it has a 100% amino acid score. Whey protein contains 114% of the essential amino acids, exceeding the value of casein. Soy is the closest plant-based amino acid score at 99%, and wheat gluten is just 25%, indicating that wheat gluten is a relatively poor protein source. The protein efficiency ratio is based on the weight gained following protein administration. This method is usually used to assess protein quality for laboratory experimentation rather than for performance applications. The biological value represents the percentage of protein incorporated into the cellular structure following ingestion. Again, in looking at this method, we see that animal protein sources score higher than plant-based protein ones. For example, whey protein has a 100% biological value, and soy protein has a 74% biological value. Regarding biological value, we see beef as less than ideal compared to others in this protein measurement system. Protein digestibility is measured by percent and represents the amount of protein the body digests. This is an important consideration as it considers a functional measurement of how a person will utilize the protein rather than just the amino acids score. The protein digestibility corrected amino acid score, or PDCAAS represents the combination of the amino acid score and the digestibility percentage, providing input that accounts for both metrics. This score has a maximum rating of 100%; therefore, several protein sources have a PDCAAS of 100%. One important thing to note is that soy protein becomes on par with many when we look at the combination of digestibility and the amino acid score. This makes soy protein an important protein source for vegetarians and vegans. The digestible indispensable amino acid score represents the amino acid score of all proteins absorbed before the distal ileum. It is this score, commonly referred to as DIAAS, where we are beginning to see the most significant level of accuracy. This score lets us know how much of the protein is digested and its digestion at a usable location. In other words, we are less concerned about digestion post distal ileum [7]. Using this score, we see that the values of individual proteins change once we factor in distal ileal digestion. Many of the sources differ from those of the PDCAAS. For example, soy protein isolate is lower as a percentage in the DIAAS but still higher than all other plant-based proteins. Milk protein or casein now has a higher score when compared to whey protein. It is important to note that whey protein has been the leader in most measures of protein quality. If we look at whey protein itself, there is also a difference in the digestible indispensable amino acid score when looking at whey protein concentrate vs whey protein isolate. This has much to do with the purity of whey protein isolate, which is 90 or higher percent compared to whey protein concentrate, which can be much less pure. This is an example of something worth considering when supplementing with protein. As we can see from the examination of the different protein rating systems, it would be incomplete to only evaluate a protein source simply by the grams of protein per ounce. The protein source's quality, digestibility, and completeness must be considered among many factors. Often in the literature, we see whey protein as the gold standard when looking at supplementation. Part of the reason, as we have seen, for this is the high performance that whey protein has in most quality-based outcomes. We also see soy protein held out as the standard in conversations regarding supplementation for vegetarian and vegan athletes; again, this has to do with the high performance of soy protein in measurements of quality when compared to other plant-based sources. Personal preference and other factors such as digestive concerns, food intolerance, or allergens must also be considered when determining protein sources.

4.3.2 Nitrogen Balance

Nitrogen balance is important for athletes in relation to their ideal protein intake for recovery and performance. It can best be visualized as a see-saw with protein taken in on one side and protein used on the other. As long as both sides are equal, the see-saw will be in balance, but as soon as one side is larger than the other, there will be an imbalance. If, for example, the amount of protein that is taken in is less than the amount that is needed, then the athlete will not be able to recover and progress in their sport. This will lead to, among other issues, the catabolism of muscle. This would be referred to as a negative nitrogen balance. If the athlete were to be taking in more protein than they need they would be able to meet the needs for their recovery and performance. This would be called positive nitrogen balance. In the ideal scenario, the athlete would have a perfectly neutral nitrogen balance, meeting their needs for performance without exceeding it. Excess protein can be stored as body fat and, in a calorically balanced diet, can replace macronutrients that may be more beneficial to the athlete, assuming they have a defined macronutrient plan. In a laboratory environment, both urine and fecal studies can be used to determine nitrogen balance, but in a clinical setting, a more clinical approach based on the defined protein needs of specific athletes may be the best approach. This approach runs the risk of being either positively or negatively balanced, so the athlete must be monitored and alterations to the diet made as needed.

4.3.3 Protein and Health

The problems associated with overeating protein are not as common as those found with other macronutrients. This is not because there are no negative effects of overeating protein but rather because it is much less common for someone to eat too much protein to see the negative effects. As with other macronutrients protein can be eaten more than the daily needs of the athlete. Excess protein can be used by the body as an energy source, although an inefficient one, to fuel the activities of daily life and performance. Additionally, excess protein can be stored by the body as body fat, which can lead to the chronic health issues associated with excess weight and obesity. I would not say that it is highly unlikely that any athlete is going to be eating enough protein to become obese, but it is possible. Some of the side effects of overeating protein include gastrointestinal dysfunction leading to both constipation and diarrhea, dehydration, increased cancer risk, increased cardiovascular disease risk, and increased liver and kidney issues due to the difficulty in processing the protein [2, 8]. Many of these conditions are worsened for older athletes who may already have some health issues that could be exacerbated. Although it is unlikely for an athlete to overconsume protein to the level of potential negative impact, it is important that the athlete or their nutritional coach make sure to focus their protein consumption on their individual needs based on the sport they compete in and the training conditions they will experience. Low protein intake is a larger concern for the health of both individuals and athletes. Adding protein into the diet can be a challenge for athletes in general and older athletes in particular. As mentioned, protein requirements for older adults are increased to support physiological functions as well as to prevent sarcopenia and other health concerns [9]. This makes it very important that older athletes need to be particularly strategic in adding protein to their diet. Simple substitutions or additions can be made to make it easier to add protein to the diet. Because food choice is highly personal, my biggest suggestions for adding protein to the diet are prioritizing protein at every meal, never eating a meal or snack without protein, and tracking your macronutrients. Prioritizing protein at meals means that if you get full, you will have gotten the protein first before any other macronutrient. This helps to ensure you get enough protein in the diet and may help to offset other calorie sources (in other words, you are not filling up on bread at dinner if you are eating your steak first). Choosing protein with all snacks does not exclude other macronutrients but helps to support the importance of protein and can help to balance out the insulin response associated with a more carbohydrate-heavy snack. Examples include an apple with peanut butter rather than just an apple, nuts and fruit instead of just fruit, a cheese stick rather than chips, etc. Finally tracking macronutrients is a necessity in the initial phases of performance eating as the connection between food choices and the actual nutrient breakdown needs to be monitored until such time as you can learn how to intuitively monitor dietary consumption. That being said, I recommend always recording your consumption even if you do not hit your goals for the day. I feel it is essential to focus your strategy by writing your planned meals and then what you actually ate at the end of the day if you want to truly maximize your results.

4.3.4 Protein Requirements

Protein is a necessary nutrient involved in muscle repair and growth. In prolonged exercise, protein is also used to fuel performance as an energy source. For these reasons, athletes need adequate protein for optimal performance. This need differs between athletes based on a variety of factors. Age, sex, lean body mass, and specific athletic requirements are all important considerations when determining protein requirements. The athlete's size, for example, is a critical consideration in deciding protein needs. A larger athlete will typically have a greater muscle mass when compared to a smaller athlete with similar body composition. Accordingly, this larger muscle mass will require more protein to recover from exercise. It, therefore, stands to reason that body size will play an important role. Sex is an important characteristic to consider when determining protein needs, this is related to both body composition and hormonal differences. Females often have a greater body fat percentage and lower lean body mass than similarly sized males. For this reason, there is an approximate 10% reduction in protein requirements for females based on their sex. Another important consideration in determining protein needs for athletes is the type of sport the athlete plays. Different sports have differing impacts on protein needs due to the muscle repair and recovery requirements and the potential use of protein as an energy source. This is due to various reasons, including the type and intensity of the sport involved. A weightlifter, for example, is constantly breaking down and repairing muscle tissue as part of their regular training regime. A more endurance-based athlete may place different stresses on the body; in this case, the duration of the activity will also impact the stressors placed on the body and protein requirements. In these sports, not only is there a breakdown in muscle tissue from the physical activity, but after the 50-minute mark, there is often a use of protein for fueling energy requirements. The intensity of the athlete's training phase should also be considered in relation to protein requirements. It is rare for an athlete to go through an entire year without variations in training intensity. Programs change throughout the year. A football player, for example, will have a different training schedule in the off-season compared to their in-season schedule. These changes may be in the type and duration of training. The differences in training plans at various times will impact the protein requirements for the athlete. The following chart discusses protein requirements for athletes engaging in different intensities of physical activities (Figure 4.3). Some interesting observations, looking at different protein requirements, are that the requirement for endurance-based athletes, for example, athletes who engage in long-duration, lower-intensity aerobic sports, are different based on the level of the athlete. Elite endurance athletes require an increased amount of protein when compared to a more moderate or even recreational endurance athlete. Conversely, when we look at resistance athletes, these are athletes who engage in strength training or other strength-related sports, we see a decline in protein requirements the longer an athlete competes in the sport. This primarily concerns the fact that in the early phases of strength sports, tremendous growth and development are seen as the athlete adapts to the new training. The speed of growth and development in strength sports slows down the longer one is involved in their given sport. For this reason, we often see strength athletes have less of a need for protein in their diet after they have competed for a significant amount of time. According to the International Society of Sports Nutrition,

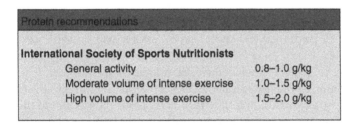

Figure 4.3 Recommended requirements for dietary protein according to the ISSN. *Source:* Potgieter [6] and Jäger et al. [10].

in their 2014 position statement, athletes looking to maintain or build muscle mass must get between 1.4 and 2.0 g of protein per kilogram of body weight daily (see Figure 4.3) [6, 10]. These numbers are slightly higher than some recommendations by other organizations, but they still fall within the AMDR for those athletes. The International Society of Sports Nutrition also noted that if the primary goal is improving body composition, slightly higher amounts of protein, over 3 g/kg of body weight per day, will promote fat mass loss while maintaining lean body mass. Bodybuilding is a sport where the primary metric of performance is aesthetics. In this case, maintaining large amounts of muscle while reducing body fat to minimal levels is desirable. This sport aims to improve body composition, so a higher protein requirement has a performance benefit.

4.3.5 Protein Requirements for Older Athletes

Master's athletes, those over the age of 35, must maintain muscle mass to recover from their chosen sport. Physiologically, after the age of 35, there is a decrease in testosterone and growth hormone, which can negatively impact nitrogen balance. It is, therefore, essential that these athletes need to ensure enough protein in their diet. As we examine the caloric requirements of master's athletes, we often see a decline in caloric needs as we age. This is due, in large part, to decreases in lean body mass. As we age, there is a need to increase protein requirements to limit or counter this decrease in lean body mass. In addition to the need for increased protein overall. To stave off some of the impacts of aging and enhance muscle protein synthesis, it is also essential that we consider the consumption of protein throughout the day. It is recommended that the athlete should aim for a minimum of 25 g of protein per meal if they are eating five meals a day or 40 g of protein per meal if they eat three meals daily [9].

4.4 Fat (Lipids)

Dietary fats, also referred to as lipids, are essential nutrients to be included in the diet both for the general public and athletes. They have many functions, including fat-soluble vitamin and hormone production, providing components of cell membranes, participating in nerve conduction, and serving as an energy source at rest and during light- to moderate-intensity exercises. The inclusion of fat in the diet is important for the athlete to be able to function in their sporting events.

Dietary fats are organic molecules containing carbon, similar to the other macronutrients. Dietary fats consist of a glycerol backbone and up to three fatty acids. Dietary fats have a hydrophobic or water-fearing end and another end that is hydrophilic or water-loving. This is where we can get separation between water and oil, imagine a drop of oil in water. The fact that fats are not water-soluble affects how they are digested, absorbed, and transported throughout the body compared to other nutrients such as carbohydrates and proteins [2]. Calorically lipids provide 9 calories/g compared to 4 calories/g of protein. This caloric density means they can provide more energy per gram, but overconsumption can also be associated with a significant increase in calories. Lipids can be found in foods from animal and plant sources.

4.4.1 Dietary Fat Classifications

Dietary fats can be classified into sterols, phospholipids, and triglycerides. Of these, triglycerides make up the most common form of dietary fats. A sterol is a fat that consists of a carbon ring formation rather than the typical carbon chain seen with other fats, like triglycerides. Phospholipids are structurally made from a glycerol group attached to two fatty acid chains, a phosphate group, and an alcohol group. The Glycerol, phosphate, and alcohol groups are hydrophilic or water-loving, whereas the two fatty acid chains are hydrophobic or water-fearing. The structure of the phospholipids, with both the hydrophobic and hydrophilic ends, means that dietary fats can be both fat and water-soluble. Phospholipids constitute cell membranes of various tissues and can help to suspend other hydrophobic liquids in water. Phospholipids are found in both plants and animals. Triglycerides are the largest group of fats in the body, foods, and beverages. These commonly occurring fats are accurately classified as simple lipids. Commonly referred to as triacylglycerol, these are the most common form of fat in the human diet, making the majority of dietary fats consumed [2]. Additionally, triglycerides are the most common fat found in the human body. They are a significant energy source and can be stored primarily in adipocytes or fat cells distributed throughout the body. Triglycerides are also stored in lesser amounts in the liver and muscles, which are more readily available for energy during exercise. When people think of dietary fat, they most likely think of triglycerides. The structure of triglycerides is like a phospholipid, consisting of a glycerol backbone, but this time attached to three fatty acids. These fatty acids may differ depending on the type of triglycerides. Triglycerides are broken down for digestion and absorption into diglycerides and monoglycerides, leaving free fatty acids in the bloodstream for use. Once stripped of all three fatty acids, the glycerol backbone may be metabolized for energy or used in the liver to form blood glucose. Functionally triglycerides serve as it is a source of energy for use during rest, starvation, and low to moderate-intensity exercise. They can be a source of energy reserves in the human body, stored as body fat, and can amount to as much as 80,000–100,000 calories in a 70-kg male with 8–12% body fat [2]. Fat is an ideal source of stored energy due to its caloric density. Fats contain 9 g per 9 calories/g compared to carbohydrates and proteins with 4 calories/g. In other words, on a gram-for-gram basis, fats provide more than twice the energy. Visceral and subcutaneous fat forms a protective layer for vital organs. It acts as a thermal barrier to protect from temperature changes or can work with temperature regulation, and fats are essential for nerve conduction. Fats play a crucial role as carriers of substances into the body and within the bloodstream carrying vitamins and other phytochemicals. Fat-soluble vitamins, for example, would not be able to be absorbed in the absence of adequate dietary fat, leading to deficiencies. Fat in food provides flavor, odor, and texture to food. Fat consumption during meals can enhance a meal's satiety or feeling of fullness. Dietary fats can be found in both plant and animal sources.

4.4.2 Fatty Acids

As with carbohydrates and protein, fats must be broken down for absorption and utilization in the diet. Fats are metabolized in the form of fatty acids. Fatty acids are carbon-based molecules arranged in a chain with a carboxyl (or acid) group on one end and a methyl group on the other. The classification or naming of fatty acids is based on the chain length, number, and location of any double bonds. Fatty acids can be classified by their chain length (the number of carbon molecules). Short-chain fatty acids contain 2–4 carbons, medium-chain fatty acids contain between 6 and 10 carbons, and long-chain fatty acids contain 12 or more carbon atoms. The shorter the carbon chain, the more liquid the fat will be at room temperature and the more soluble it will be in water. Short and medium-chain fatty acids are digested and absorbed more quickly than long-chain fatty acids. Short-chain fatty acids are rarely found naturally in food except for butyric acid, which is found in milk. Most short-chain fatty acids are a byproduct of bacterial fermentation in the large intestine.

4.4.3 Saturated or Unsaturated Fats

Examination of the chemical structure of fatty acids shows that all carbon atoms participate in four bonds. In saturated fats, all carbons join in a single

> **Potential health implications of trans-fats**
>
> Increased inflammatory biomarkers (TNF, IL-6, CRP)
> Dyslipidemia biomarkers (increased LDLs, apo-B decreased HDLs)
> Increased insulin resistance (increased obesity and visceral fat)
> Coronary heart disease

Figure 4.4 Health concerns associated with dietary trans fats. *Source:* Adapted from Gropper and Smith [2].

bond with another carbon or hydrogen. In monounsaturated fat, one of those carbon-to-carbon bonds will be a double bond; in polyunsaturated fat, there are two or more double bonds in the carbon chain. Hydrogenation refers to the process of adding hydrogen atoms to unsaturated fat to convert it to saturated fat. This process is used for foods in which the properties of saturated fat are preferred or the saturated fat is unavailable. One example of this is the creation of margarine from oil. Margarine was created at a time when butter was being rationed. Margarine was developed by hydrogenating oil to create a solid product that was flavored to look, feel, and taste like butter. This hydrogenation process resulted in the formation of trans fatty acids, which have potentially harmful health implications (see Figure 4.4) [2].

4.4.4 Omega-3 and -6 Fatty Acids

The methyl end of a fatty acid is also called the omega end. The double bond that occurs closest to this end identifies the classification of the fatty acid. Because of this, we know that omega fatty acids are all unsaturated fatty acids and will contain a double bond. Omega-3 fatty acids will have the first double bond at the third carbon, and omega-6 fatty acids will have the double bond at the sixth carbon. An omega fatty acid may contain more than one double bond, but the name only shows where the first one is. Omega-3 fatty acids form localized hormones known as eicosanoids, which can dilate blood vessels, reduce inflammation, reduce blood clotting, and carry health benefits [11]. In contrast, omega-6 fatty acids promote the inflammatory process, which can increase blood clotting, leading to vasoconstriction, and potentially have negative health implications.

4.4.5 Essential Fatty Acids

Much like our conversation about protein, fatty acids can be classified as either essential or nonessential. Nonessential fatty acids can be produced from other sources and are not required from the diet. Essential fatty acids cannot be produced internally and must be consumed as part of the diet or taken in supplement form. Linoleic and linolenic acid are both considered essential fatty acids.

4.4.6 Ketogenic Diets and Performance

The discussion of macronutrient needs for performance would only be complete with, at least partially, discussing athletes' use of a ketogenic diet. A ketogenic diet will be focused on the use of ketogenesis for the production of energy from dietary fats and not from carbohydrates. The two main characteristics of the diet are that the dietary consumption of carbohydrates is traditionally kept to less than 5% of the total caloric intake (e.g., 100 calories or 25 g on a 2000-calorie diet). Total fat intake will be approximately 70% of the total caloric intake (e.g., 1400 calories or ~156 g on a 2000 calorie diet). The remaining 25% of the calories for the ketogenic diet would come from protein consumption (e.g., 500 calories or 125 g on a 2000-calorie diet). In this diet, energy comes primarily from the production and use of ketone bodies. Still, after adaptation to the diet (which can take a year for complete keto-adaptation), glycogen production is identical to that of a mixed diet, as identified by Volek et al. [12]. This type of diet will be ideal for athletes who use either stored glycogen to fuel performance or for athletes using lower-intensity exercise and can bypass the use of carbohydrates as the primary energy source for performance. Volek et al. noted that the fully keto-adapted athlete would replenish glycogen as quickly as a non-keto-adapted athlete and increase the intensity at which they can oxidize fat to fuel performance [12]. This would indicate that for a fully keto-adapted athlete, energy will be maintained at a higher intensity level. This would increase the applicability of this diet to more types of sports. Some benefits of a diet of this type for an athlete would be regulating blood sugar and the ready availability of a much larger energy source (reducing some of the need for intra-workout nutrition). Some of the negatives surrounding this diet are primarily in the difficulty that some will have to maintain the diet and the speed with which even a tiny overconsumption of carbohydrates will have on the adaptive state. Additionally, some athletes and some sports will favor a diet higher in carbohydrates for performance. A strength athlete may use a ketogenic diet, for example, to control their body weight or lose body fat before a contest. Still, they may perform better with added dietary carbohydrates when trying to add muscle or in a strength accumulation phase of training. Common misconceptions are that the diet cannot be healthy due to the large amount of fat needed to maintain the diet, the diet cannot be used by athletes as carbohydrates are the primary source of energy for the athlete, and a ketogenic diet requires too much protein. These misconceptions are not fact-based, as research has shown that adherents to a ketogenic diet often see improvements in blood biomarkers, such as those for cardiovascular disease. As mentioned earlier, the body can use alternative sources to fuel performance through fat oxidation with minimal loss in performance [12].

The masters athlete may consider the use of a ketogenic diet for a variety of reasons. First, as the athlete ages, there is a decrease in insulin sensitivity, which can predispose the athlete to some common chronic health concerns such as diabetes, weight gain, and systemic inflammation. A ketogenic diet would reduce some of this impact as insulin sensitivity has been shown to increase with the initiation of a ketogenic diet. As the metabolism slows with age, the athlete tends to put on excess weight more quickly. Athletes consuming a ketogenic diet are less likely to gain weight as a fully keto-adapted individual has a decreased average caloric consumption overall. This does not mean that a keto-adapted athlete cannot overdue consumption; instead, it is less likely that they will. Finally, there are some evidence of hormonal benefits for the keto-adapted individual, which may be favorable for the older athlete as there is an increase in some of the hormones that would typically decline with age, although the research is not consistent with this [13]. This is not to say that a ketogenic diet will work for every older athlete or should be used by all masters athletes. Instead, it would be worth considering for the athlete looking for an alternate approach to their performance diet.

4.5 Conclusion

The primary source of the fuel the athlete needs to perform athletically and recover from training and competition comes from the macronutrients in their diet. The dietary macronutrients carbohydrates, protein, and fats comprise the athlete's diet's calorie-containing portion. Carbohydrates provide the athlete with fuel for performance and cellular functions. These nutrients are essential for higher-intensity athletics and provide the first source of ATP for activities. Proteins provide the body with structural and functional purposes, from the makeup of the muscular system to the production of the enzymes needed for many biochemical processes needed for homeostatic balance. Dietary protein can also serve as a source of energy in some circumstances. Fats are essential and function to produce hormones, absorb vitamins, support the nervous system, act as a storage form of energy, as well as, assist in thermoregulation. These three nutrients work in tandem to support homeostatic balance for the athlete as well as to provide the substrate needed for them to perform and recover to their maximal capacity.

References

1. Cermak NM, van Loon LJ. The use of carbohydrates during exercise as an ergogenic aid. *Sports Med.* 2013;43(11):1139-1155. doi:10.1007/s40279-013-0079-0
2. Gropper SS, Smith JL. *Advanced Nutrition and Human Metabolism.* Cengage Learning, 2018.
3. Manore MM. Exercise and the Institute of Medicine recommendations for nutrition. *Curr. Sports Med. Rep.* 2005;4(4):193-198. doi:10.1097/01.csmr.0000306206.72186.00
4. Siri PW, Krauss RM. Influence of dietary carbohydrate and fat on LDL and HDL particle distributions. *Curr. Atheroscler. Rep.* 2005;7(6):455-459. doi:10.1007/s11883-005-0062-9
5. Tungare S, Paranjpe AG. *Diet and Nutrition to Prevent Dental Problems.* [Updated 2023 Jul 10]. In: StatPearls [Internet]. Treasure Island (FL): StatPearls Publishing, 2024. Available from: https://www.ncbi.nlm.nih.gov/books/NBK534248/
6. Potgieter S. Sport nutrition: a review of the latest guidelines for exercise and sport nutrition from the American College of Sport Nutrition, the International Olympic Committee and the International Society for Sports Nutrition. *South Afr. J. Clin. Nutr.* 2013;26(1):6-16.
7. Adhikari S, Schop M, de Boer IJ, Huppertz T. Protein quality in perspective: a review of protein quality metrics and their applications. *Nutrients* 2022;14(5):947.
8. Delimaris I. Adverse effects associated with protein intake above the recommended dietary allowance for adults. *ISRN Nutr.* 2013;2013:126929. Published 2013 Jul 18. doi:10.5402/2013/126929
9. Baum JI, Kim IY, Wolfe RR. Protein consumption and the elderly: what is the optimal level of intake?. *Nutrients.* 2016;8(6):359. Published 2016 Jun 8. doi:10.3390/nu8060359
10. Jäger R, Kerksick CM, Campbell BI, et al. International Society of Sports Nutrition Position Stand: protein and exercise. *J. Int. Soc. Sports Nutr.* 2017;14:20. Published 2017 Jun 20. doi:10.1186/s12970-017-0177-8
11. Shahidi F, Ambigaipalan P. Omega-3 polyunsaturated fatty acids and their health benefits. *Annu. Rev. Food Sci. Technol.* 2018;9:345-381. doi:10.1146/annurev-food-111317-095850
12. Volek JS, Freidenreich DJ, Saenz C, et al. Metabolic characteristics of keto-adapted ultra-endurance runners. *Metabolism.* 2016;65(3):100-110.
13. Wilson JM, Lowery RP, Roberts MD, et al. Effects of ketogenic dieting on body composition, strength, power, and hormonal profiles in resistance training men. *J. Strength Cond. Res.* 2020;34(12):3463-3474.

5

Micronutrients

5.1 Introduction

The term micronutrient refers to the nutrients, specifically the vitamins and minerals, that we need in small amounts to carry out the functions needed to maintain the homeostatic balance of the individual. These nutrients are required in smaller quantities which is different from the macronutrients that must be consumed in more significant quantities. Although required in smaller doses, they are still essential to human beings functioning as part of biochemical processes such as energy production, wound healing, growth and development, and DNA repair. In most cases, our bodies can either not synthesize the micronutrient or not synthesize them in adequate amounts to survive. These micronutrients do not supply energy and do not contain calories. Even though they do not provide energy, as macronutrients do, they are no less essential to vital functions. Let us look at energy, for example, as previously mentioned micronutrients do not directly provide energy in the form of calories, but serve as coenzymes in metabolizing macronutrients to produce energy. Therefore, we need micronutrients in adequate amounts as part of the process of energy production. In this chapter, micronutrients will be presented by looking at their functionality, requirements, deficiencies, toxicities, clinical applications, and food sources.

5.2 Vitamin Overview

Why are vitamins given the name vitamin? The etymology of the term vitamin is important as it helps shine a light on their value in health and performance. The term vitamin is derived from the terms vital and amine.

Sports Nutrition for Masters Athletes, First Edition. Peter G. Nickless.
© 2025 John Wiley & Sons, Inc. Published 2025 by John Wiley & Sons, Inc.

The reason was that the first vitamins discovered contained amine groups (NH_3) and were considered vital to life. Therefore, these newly discovered compounds were considered vital amines or simply vitamins [1]. As time passed, we found that not all vitamins contain amine groups, but the name vitamin has stuck.

All vitamins are organic compounds. Organic compounds are those that contain carbon. One aspect of these compounds is that sometimes they are less stable when compared to inorganic compounds, meaning that they can be damaged or destroyed depending on a range of factors. Heat or cold, for example, could destroy specific vitamins rendering them less bioavailable to carry on their functions. How we prepare the foods that we eat in another way can impact the vitamins found within the food and their impacts on the bodily processes involved. Boiling, for example, can reduce the amount of riboflavin contained in foods.

Vitamins are categorized based on their solubility in different media as they follow different routes through digestion and absorption and have differences in the way that they are transported to tissues. The storage of vitamins has differences as well. Some vitamins are fat-soluble, while the majority of vitamins, in terms of different types, are soluble in water. Fat-soluble and water-soluble vitamins differ in digestion and absorption, transport, and storage, as well as the likelihood of developing toxicity if an excess amount is taken [1]. Water-soluble vitamins do not reach toxic levels as easily, for example, and can be taken in higher dosages with less potential negative impact. The downside to water-soluble vitamins is that they are generally not stored if taken in excess. The fat-soluble vitamins on the other hand can be stored in the body but, unfortunately, can reach a toxic level and intake must be controlled to limit toxicity. The study of vitamins involves learning about each vitamin separately. This is because, although categorized as a group, they each will have differences in their physiological roles, each of which should be examined and understood. Fatty acids, for example, share standard features and are chemically related; however, vitamins B1 and B2 are not.

5.2.1 Water-Soluble Vitamins

Water-soluble vitamins can be absorbed directly into the bloodstream and do not require lipoproteins to carry them around. Unfortunately, water-soluble vitamins cannot be retained for long periods in the body, although some can be stored longer than others, for example, vitamin B12. Storage occurs only when the vitamin is bound to enzymes or transport proteins [1]. Any excess consumption of water-soluble vitamins is excreted in urine. The lack of storage ability means that we must ensure adequate daily intake

Vitamin C (ascorbic acid)	
Thiamin (B1)	Vitamin B6
Riboflavin (B2)	Biotin
Niacin (B3)	Folate
Pantothenic acid (B5)	Vitamin B12 (Cobalamin)

Figure 5.1 Water-soluble vitamins.

to account for water-soluble vitamins that have been lost or used. The only way to save these vitamins is to put them into action by converting them into their active coenzyme form. These vitamins participate in a variety of reactions, including energy-releasing reactions, immune support, protein synthesis, and blood cell formation (Figure 5.1).

5.2.2 Fat-Soluble Vitamins

Fat-soluble vitamins (A, D, E, and K), unlike water-soluble vitamins, do not enter directly into the bloodstream but first must cross the brush border before entering the intestinal cells. They then can enter the lymphatic vessels as a type of lipoprotein called a chylomicron. A chylomicron is a particle that carries dietary lipids. Simply put, fat-soluble vitamins do not enter the bloodstream directly but are carried by the lymphatic vessel to the bloodstream first [1]. Water-soluble vitamins (all B and C vitamins) have no trouble traveling across intestinal cells and into the bloodstream directly and can then be carried around the body.

Vitamins A, D, E, and K are similar to other dietary lipids. They dissolve in fat and are usually absorbed at the same time and manner as when other fat absorption occurs. They need bile salts as an emulsifier. An emulsifier is a substance that can help oil and water to mix. Anything that interferes with the normal process of lipid absorption will interfere with the absorption of fat-soluble vitamins. If you have a fat absorption issue or do not have much fat in your diet, the digestion of these fat-soluble vitamins could be compromised. Athletes who consume low-fat diets can see problems with the amounts of fat-soluble vitamins they get from their diet. Following absorption, fat-soluble vitamins are transported like other nonpolar lipids in lipoproteins inside chylomicrons. These chylomicrons carry dietary lipids as well. Fat-soluble vitamins have the distinction of being able to be stored in the body. These vitamins are stored in the lipid fraction inside the cells and can be found in large amounts in the liver [1]. With high consumption, fat-soluble vitamins can accumulate in the body and develop toxicity, the impacts of which will vary depending on the type of vitamin (Figure 5.2).

Vitamin A	Vitamin E
Vitamin D	Vitamin K

Figure 5.2 Fat-soluble vitamins.

Calcium	Phosphorus	Sulfur
Chloride	Potassium	
Magnesium	Sodium	

Figure 5.3 Major minerals.

5.2.3 Major Minerals

The classification of major minerals includes minerals that the human body uses in larger quantities. Although the body can store these minerals, it does not produce them, so they must be included in the diet. Calcium, chloride, magnesium, phosphorus, potassium, sodium, and sulfur are included as major minerals (Figure 5.3).

5.2.4 Electrolytes

The electrolytes sodium, calcium, chloride, magnesium, and potassium function to assist the athlete in carrying on vital processes in the body. The functions of electrolytes include fluid balance, maintaining cellular neutrality, and a vital role in action potentials in nerves and muscles. These elements are essential as they are required in the diet as they cannot be produced by the body. Electrolytes must be kept in balance as extreme deviations can lead to potentially deadly health issues (Figure 5.4).

5.2.5 Essential Trace Minerals

Essential trace minerals are those minerals that are needed by the body in smaller amounts. They are vital for the function of the body, and they cannot be produced internally, so they must be consumed as part of the diet. The essential trace elements include chromium, copper, iodine, iron, manganese, molybdenum, selenium, and zinc. Functionally, these minerals are catalysts in enzyme systems, participate in oxidation–reduction reactions, and as participate in the transportation of iron (Figure 5.5).

Sodium	Calcium
Potassium	Magnesium
Chloride	

Figure 5.4 Electrolytes.

Iron	Chromium
Zinc	Iodine
Copper	Manganese
Selenium	Molybdenum

Figure 5.5 Essential trace minerals.

5.2.6 Nonessential Trace Minerals

The classification nonessential trace minerals are minerals that are not required in large quantities and are not required to be eaten to carry out vital functions. These minerals are functionally active but are not required in and particular amount

Fluoride	Silicon
Arsenic	Vanadium
Boron	Cobalt
Nickel	

Figure 5.6 Nonessential trace minerals.

in the diet and, therefore, have no established RDA. These minerals include arsenic, boron, fluoride, nickel, silicon, cobalt, and vanadium (Figure 5.6).

5.3 Dietary Reference Intakes

We eat food for many reasons pleasure, function, social reasons, etc. Food is required because it contains the nutrients needed for our bodies to function. Nutrients are the chemicals and compounds that our body uses for growth, development, athletic performance, and maintaining health. Many of these nutrients are considered to be essential. Essential nutrients cannot be produced in our body. Therefore, we must get these essential nutrients from our diet. For humans to maintain health, we need the right food combinations to get the nutrients to support optimum function. At different stages in our lives, the requirements for specific nutrients change. Many factors can affect the need for essential nutrients. Age, for example, can impact the nutrients needed. Consider how fast a baby grows; compare this to someone over 80. They have different nutrient needs due to the changes their bodies are undergoing. Differing levels of physical activity or even employment will have different requirements for nutrients, and what is adequate for one person may not be adequate for another. Think about the early stages in life, shortly after birth or during our first growth spurt; where do all the extra minerals for bone, muscle, and connective tissue come from? They come from our diet. Two identical people, one in a healthy state and one with an illness, will have different needs. Athletic participation will also require other nutrients based on the sport and duration of activity. If you do not provide enough energy for your body to recover, it will be harder for you to recover from athletics and rebuild. Lifestyle habits (such as smoking, stress, or alcohol abuse) can influence metabolism and nutrient requirements. If we abuse alcohol, our bodies will need many more vitamins to maintain healthy function for various reasons. There are even diseases that are related to alcohol's impact on a B vitamin deficiency. During pregnancy, the mother must increase her eating as a child grows in her uterus. During this stage, the requirements for many essential nutrients will increase. Dietary intake standards were developed for the public. They cannot account for all the factors that may impact a person, but they do account for age, gender, growth, pregnancy, and lactation.

Dietary reference intakes are the standards developed for healthy people at different stages of life. Keep that in mind that they are not intended to take athletics into account, and therefore, while essential to discuss, the needs of athletes will often be larger than the intake standards for some specific nutrients. The Food and Nutrition Board of the National Academies of Sciences Engineering and Medicine develops them based on available scientific evidence [2].

There are four elements of Dietary Reference Intake (DRI):

1) **Estimated average requirement** (EAR) – is the amount of a nutrient that would meet the needed intake for half of the population in a specific life stage and gender group. The EAR is used to assess the adequacy of intakes for population groups. EAR requires scientific evidence [2].
2) **Recommended daily allowance** (RDA) – is the amount of a nutrient that will meet the needs of most healthy people (97–98%) in a specific life stage and gender group while decreasing the risk for certain chronic diseases. The RDA is calculated as EAR + 2 statistical standard deviations. Some nutrients do not have an RDA which is often due to a lack of the scientific evidence needed to establish one. The RDA is calculated based on EAR, so if there is not enough evidence to establish an EAR, there will not be enough for an RDA. The RDA is a calculated number based on probability. Therefore, a dietary intake level at or close to the RDA is very likely, but not guaranteed, to meet the needs of a specific population. Population estimates like this are best used for group analysis or as a baseline, but not as the only determination of an individual's needs. An individual's actual needs must consider the various factors previously discussed. Athletes will often, but not always, have needs that will be more than the established RDAs for the age and sex groups. As we discuss the functions of the individual nutrients, we will better understand how their need for these functions will increase for athletes and, accordingly, the nutrient needs will increase [2].
3) **Adequate intake** (AI) – is considered a tentative RDA. It is used for nutrients that do not have sufficient evidence to establish an RDA. In this case, an AI can be formulated even though an RDA cannot be established. The AI is the amount estimated to be adequate for most people. An AI is used when the scientific community does not have enough evidence to develop an RDA but enough to make recommendations [2].

4) **Tolerable upper intake levels** (ULs) – represent the upper limits of intake before the user may potentially experience adverse effects. The UL does not reflect the desired intake level; instead, it means the total level of daily intake that should be kept within the maximum. This would include the total daily intake of foods, fortified foods, and supplements. Exceeding the UL for a nutrient, if established, could result in toxicity and side effects. A diet rich in whole foods is less likely to reach toxicity compared to supplements. This is often due to the amounts of a nutrient being significantly more in a supplement vs in a food. Although the UL is often best to avoid, some studies suggest the UL may increase based on the individual's presentation [2].

As mentioned, these DRIs do not consider the needs of the individual. Still, they are derived from population studies and must be used differently for a population vs an individual. A population will use the DRI to assess the adequacy of intake and see if the population group is taking in adequate nutrients or is at risk for deficiency. This is ideal when conducting research or evaluation of a group of people. If I were evaluating the eating habits of a school in general, looking to see if the students were consuming the DRIs for their age group would give me insight into their nutritional status in general but not specifically if one student is recovering from their activities. Population group information can be used to plan diets for large groups and set policies and guidelines to avoid deficiency but have less value for the individual. Individuals can use the RDA and AIs as targets for minimum intake. Some nutrients must be consumed more than the RDA and the AIs for special populations, like older athletes, and must be evaluated individually. The best use of these DRIs is preventing deficiency, not a performance optimization. As the UL can carry side effects, care must be taken to stay away from the UL level for the nutrients, for the most part.

5.3.1 Limitations of the DRI

The DRIs are developed and updated based on available scientific evidence, but we are still doing much learning when it comes to the human body. This means that DRIs will change as new scientific evidence becomes available concerning the nutrition of a micronutrient and its relationship with health. There needs to be significant scientific evidence to reach a point where we can make recommendations to change DRIs. In 2011, for example, the DRIs were updated regarding recommendations for calcium and Vitamin D [3]. Enough scientific research has been done on these nutrients to feel comfortable making changes to the DRIs. The primary use of DRIs is to maintain health and reduce the risk of certain diseases. This is because DRIs are developed to maintain health and avoid diseases or conditions associated with deficiency. To achieve optimal health and or performance or to achieve the health of a sick person, the DRI may need to be exceeded, and, ideally, the needs for nutrients should be determined individually based on a personalized approach. Determining the DRI needs of an individual should consider things like physical activity, smoking, environmental stressors, etc., to customize a strategy to micronutrient recommendations.

5.3.2 Fortification vs Enrichment

Fortification is the addition of nutrients to foods that may not be present in the food, to begin with. For example, milk is fortified with vitamin D to help your body absorb the calcium. Since Vitamin D is necessary for calcium absorption, adding Vitamin D to milk makes sense to help with calcium absorption. Enrichment, on the other hand, is the addition of nutrients lost during food processing. For example, B vitamins lost when wheat is refined are added back to white flour. Enriching foods back to their original content would not be feasible compared to unprocessed food, so enriched foods often carry a different micronutrient content than their nonenriched counterparts. Fortification and enrichment of foods have been an effective means of ensuring specific macronutrient needs are met, at a population level, for people who may be consuming more processed than whole foods.

5.4 Water-Soluble Vitamins

The category of water-soluble vitamins consists of vitamins, eight of which are identified as B vitamins. Vitamin C, or ascorbic acid, is the only water-soluble vitamin not in the B vitamin family. Functionally, most of these vitamins will fall into one of two categories. The first category of water-soluble vitamins is energy-releasing vitamins. The second category participates in hematopoietic (or blood cell-producing) reactions. These categories comprise the majority, but not all, of the functions of water-soluble vitamins. Many of the water-soluble vitamins will have multiple effects functionally and will fit into more than one category. One example of this is vitamin B6, which carries hematopoietic and energy production functions in addition to other functions. Vitamins are often named by their common name, chemical name, and coenzyme name. These can be confusing, but they are all important to know as we discuss water-soluble vitamins in more detail. Any nutritional professional looking to work with an athlete's micronutrient needs should know all three names and the functions of all vitamins. However, the common name functionally will be used in working with athletes.

5.4.1 Vitamin B1

Vitamin B1 is also referred to by the chemical name of thiamine and the coenzyme name of thiamine pyrophosphate. Thiamine has functions that include roles as a coenzyme in energy production, the transmission of nerve impulses, the production of neurotransmitters, and the synthesis of the protein collagen. Thiamine deficiency can result in altered sensation in the extremities, gait and balance disturbance, confusion and learning difficulties, headaches, depression, irritability, muscle tenderness, anemia, cardiovascular issues, fatigue, poor wound healing, reduced immunity, loss of appetite, and constipation. Some groups are more likely to see deficiencies in thiamine and include those with increased alcohol consumption, older adults due to decreases in food consumption, those with folate deficiency, those who consume substantial amounts of coffee and black tea, and those who consume higher amounts of processed foods that are unenriched. The RDA of thiamine is 1.2 mg for men and 1.1 mg for women. There is an increase in requirements for thiamine seen for pregnant or lactating women, those with diseases associated with malabsorption, and those with increased physiological stressors. The RDA rises to 1.4 mg for pregnant and lactating women. There is no current UL noted for thiamine, and it is nontoxic. Thiamine is not stored in the body; therefore, daily consumption of the DRI is vital to avoid deficiency. Therapeutically, thiamine has been used to treat neuropathy, Alzheimer's disease, anxiety, depression, heart failure, and anemia. Due to their increased physiological demands, athletes may see an increased need for thiamine to support optimal performance if dietary consumption or absorption is less than adequate. Food sources for thiamin are widespread and include sources from both plants and animals. Plant sources of thiamin include brewer's yeast, oatmeal, sunflower seeds, wheat germ, legumes, soy milk, peas, and potatoes. Animal sources include meats, particularly pork and salmon. Additionally, processed foods are enriched with thiamine, resulting in fewer cases of deficiency due to dietary lack of consumption. Exposure to heat, as in cooking, may reduce the amount of thiamine in foods [1, 4–6].

5.4.2 Vitamin B2

The chemical name for vitamin B2 is riboflavin, but it can also be referred to by one of its two coenzyme derivative forms, flavin mononucleotide (FMN) and flavin adenine dinucleotide (FAD). The functions of riboflavin include energy production and its actions as an antioxidant. FAD and FMN function as coenzymes in the metabolism of carbohydrates, fatty acids, and proteins through support for the TCA cycle, support for beta-oxidation, the process by which fatty acids are converted to acetyl-CoA for the TCA cycle, helps to convert other B vitamins into their coenzyme form like B6, folate, niacin (B3). Riboflavin is required for the reduction of glutathione. Populations at risk for deficiency include those with large alcohol consumption, thyroid disease, diabetes mellitus, trauma, and physical and emotional stress. Female athletes will also have a higher risk of deficiency of riboflavin. Symptoms of deficiency include glossitis (inflammation of the tongue), seborrheic dermatitis (itchy, moist, scaly skin) inflammation, angular stomatitis (sores/cracking in the corner of the mouth), cheilosis (cracks and sores on the angles of the mouth), photophobia, anemia due to decreased red blood cell production, lethargy, depression, and personality changes. The RDA for riboflavin is 1.3 mg/day for males and 1.1 mg/day for females. Pregnancy will increase the RDA to 1.4 mg/day, and lactation will increase the requirement to 1.6 mg/day. No UL has been established, and no toxic or adverse effects of high riboflavin intake in humans are known. Large doses of riboflavin can lead to a bright yellow color in urine. This color change is harmless in terms of physiological impact. Clinical applications include detoxification from oxidative reduction, antioxidant functions (due to glutathione reductase activity), fatigue, depression, migraines, and skin and mucous issues. Athletic benefits of riboflavin are associated with energy production roles but are limited, with the primary use to athletes being in avoiding deficiency. This could be more of a concern for older athletic populations who see a requirement increase. Sources of riboflavin are primarily of animal origin, including dairy products, such as milk and cheese, eggs, and meat. Plant sources, although less common, include legumes and green vegetables. Refined grains are among the foods enriched with riboflavin, so deficiency is rare. Riboflavin can be destroyed by bright light (which is why milk should be stored in opaque containers), and riboflavin content can be reduced when cooking in water [1, 4, 5].

5.4.3 Vitamin B3

Vitamin B3 is known by its chemical name, niacin, and its two active compounds, nicotinic acid and nicotinamide. The functions of niacin include DNA replication and repair, blood sugar regulation, a significant coenzyme in oxidation/reduction, glycolysis, oxidative decarboxylation of pyruvate, oxidation of acetyl-CoA in the TCA cycle, fatty acid metabolism, fatty acid and cholesterol synthesis, and steroid hormone synthesis. Deficiencies in niacin can result in pellagra. Pellagra is characterized by the 4Ds dermatitis (patches of red scaly skin), dementia, diarrhea, and death. Increased risk for deficiency is noted for those with a dietary lack of niacin-containing foods (specifically those on hypo-caloric or low-protein diets), those with a vitamin B6 deficiency, diseases that would limit absorption, such as IBS, and alcoholism. The RDA for niacin is 16 mg/day for adult males and 14 mg/day for adult females. The RDA increases to 18 mg/day for pregnant women and 17 mg/day for lactating women. The term niacin equivalent (NE) was developed to find a way to equate endogenous and exogenous forms of niacin. Niacin can be synthesized in the liver from tryptophan. Intake of 1 g of high-quality (complete) protein should contain approximately 10 mg of tryptophan. Sixty milligram of tryptophan should generate 1 mg of niacin. Therefore, ingesting 6 g of high-quality protein should equal 1 mg of niacin or 1 NE. The typical diet in the United States contains ~800 mg of tryptophan daily or ~13.3 NE (not all tryptophan will be used to produce niacin as the tryptophan needs must be met first). The UL for niacin is 35 mg/day. This UL is based on supplements and fortified foods, as niacin toxicity from whole food is not known to cause toxic effects. Nicotinamide is generally better tolerated in larger doses when compared to nicotinic acid. A large dose of nicotinic acid, over 500 mg/day, could result in vasodilation-related effects of tingling and flushing. They are sometimes referred to as the "niacin flush." Over 2.5 g/day dosages can lead to headaches, gastrointestinal problems, liver injury, hyperuricemia, and glucose intolerance. Clinical applications for niacin include lowering cholesterol with nicotinic acid. Nicotinamide may be used to support those diagnosed with some mental illnesses, niacin may help reduce the degenerative changes with arthritis, nicotinamide may be beneficial for diabetes, niacin is an antioxidant that may help protect against environmental stressors, nicotinic acid may help with the prevention of headaches, and the dilatory effects of nicotinic acid may help some circulatory disorders. Food sources for niacin include beef liver, chicken, tuna from animal sources, mushrooms, and enriched rice from plant sources. Niacin is required to enrich processed foods, reducing the risk of deficiency. The niacin content of food can be reduced when cooking in water, as in boiling [1, 4, 5, 7].

5.4.4 Vitamin B5

The chemical name for vitamin B5 is pantothenic acid. The active form of pantothenic acid is coenzyme A, which is particularly important in metabolism. The functions of pantothenic acid include energy production. CoA is required for the biochemical pathways that produce energy from the macronutrients carbohydrates, proteins, and fats. Coenzyme A is involved in producing essential fatty acids, cholesterol, melatonin, acetylcholine, and heme. Coenzyme A is also necessary for metabolizing some drugs and toxins in the liver. Deficiencies in pantothenic acid are rare, but the symptoms include burning feet syndrome (burning sensation in the feet and numbness), vomiting, fatigue, and personality changes like irritability. These symptoms are nonspecific and, accordingly, often not easy to spot. Populations particularly at risk for deficiency are alcoholics, chronic illness, and heavy dieting. Deficiency in pantothenic acid is rare and often accompanies severe malnutrition, where we would see a multitude of nutritional deficiencies. The adequate intake (AI) for pantothenic acids is 5 mg/day for adult males and females. The AI for pregnant females increases to 6 mg/day, and lactating females will have an AI of 7 mg/day. There is no established UL for pantothenic acid, considered nontoxic in doses as high as 10 g. Pantothenic acid can treat microcytic anemias, acne, lupus, fatigue, arthritis, wound healing, and dyslipidemia. While athletes may find benefit to supplementation, this benefit is largely due to preventing deficiency more than performance enhancement. Dietary sources of pantothenic acid include animal sources, such as calf liver, lobster, and eggs, and plant sources, like Brewer's yeast, peanuts, peas, soybeans, watermelon, broccoli, and brown rice. Brewer's yeast can provide up to 10 g of pantothenic acid per serving [1, 4, 5, 8].

5.4.5 Vitamin B6

Vitamin B6 is known by its chemical name, pyridoxine. The active form of pyridoxine is pyridoxal-5-phosphate (PLP). This activation requires zinc and riboflavin, so deficiencies in these nutrients can impact vitamin B6 availability. The functions of pyridoxine as PLP are associated with many metabolic reactions and are involved in amino acid synthesis. Collagen, a protein essential for tissue healing and structure, depends on pyridoxine. PLP helps to maintain healthy blood sugar, supports the metabolism of homocysteine, energy production, the formation of niacin from tryptophan, lipid synthesis and metabolism (particularly lipids involved in the myelin sheath and cell membranes), hemoglobin synthesis, and neurotransmitter synthesis. Deficiencies in vitamin B6 can result in red scaly, greasy, and painful patches on the skin, angular cheilosis, anemia, reduced immune function, muscle twitching, convulsions, behavioral changes, burning and tingling in the hands and feet, and increased risk of dyslipidemia and kidney stone formation. Populations that are at an increased risk of deficiency include those with digestive disorders that impact metabolism, older individuals, people who consume high protein diets, high caffeine consumption, alcoholics, pregnant and lactating women, those who smoke, some medications such as oral contraceptives and anticonvulsants, and some chronic diseases. Female athletes are at a higher risk of deficiency of vitamin B6. The RDA for vitamin B6 for adult males and females is 1.3 mg/day, increasing to 1.5 mg/day for females and 1.7 mg/day for males over 50. Pregnant and lactating women will see their dietary needs increase to 1.9 mg/day and 2.0 mg/day, respectively. The UL for Vitamin B6 is 100 mg/day. Toxicity, while not common from whole food forms, can result in neuropathy, pain, numbness in the extremities, and difficulty walking. Clinically, vitamin B6 is used to treat skin disorders, can help with reducing food allergies, can help support asthma, can be beneficial with atherosclerosis, some anemias, morning sickness, premenstrual syndrome symptoms, support mood such as depression, arthritis, kidney stones, carpel tunnel like symptoms, epilepsy, improve immune function, and support some psychological conditions. Athletes who consume a higher protein diet must ensure they get enough vitamin B6, particularly as they age. Exercise increases the need for vitamin B6, particularly due to its role in energy production and hemopoiesis. Food sources of Vitamin B6 include calf and chicken liver, turkey, and trout from animal sources and potatoes, bananas, lentils, spinach, and Brewer's yeast from plant sources. Vitamin B6 is included in the fortification of processed foods in the United States; therefore, deficiency is uncommon. Heat, light, cooking in water (boiling), and a high fiber concentration in foods may reduce the bioavailability of B6 in foods [1, 4, 9, 10].

5.4.6 Vitamin B7

The chemical name of vitamin B7 is biotin. Although vitamin B7 and vitamin H can be used, biotin is the most common terminology. The functions of biotin include the synthesis of glucose, which requires biotin as an enzyme. Biotin is necessary as part of an enzyme for producing and metabolizing fatty acids. Biotin-containing enzymes are essential for metabolizing the amino acids threonine, isoleucine, and methionine. Biotin also is needed for its role in DNA synthesis. A biotin deficiency can result in hair loss, a scaly red rash around the mouth, eyes, and genital area, lethargy, depression, anxiety, hallucinations, seizures, developmental delays, anorexia, muscle aches, and reduced immune function. Populations with an increased risk for deficiency include pregnant and lactating, malnutrition, severe caloric restriction, eating raw eggs (avidin in raw eggs can prevent biotin absorption), and taking antibiotics and anticonvulsants. The AI for biotin is 30 μg/day for both adult males and females. Lactation will increase the AI to 35 μg/day. No UL is established for biotin, and it is considered nontoxic. A small portion of biotin is produced in the intestinal bacteria, which can help to contribute to the daily requirements. Clinically biotin has been associated with treating impaired biotin metabolism, supplemented during long-term anticonvulsant use, blood sugar control for diabetics and dermatological disorders, and treating dry and brittle hair and nails. Food sources of biotin include animal sources such as eggs, calf's liver, and milk. Plant sources of biotin include avocados, mushrooms, oatmeal, soybeans, and brewer's yeast [1, 4].

5.4.7 Folate

The active form of folate is tetrahydrofolate (THF). The functions of folate include DNA and RNA synthesis, tissue repair, protein synthesis, red blood cell production, production and the interconversion of amino acids, and fetal development (particularly the development of the central nervous system). Populations with an increased risk of folate deficiency include smokers, those in periods of rapid growth such as pregnancy, childhood, and adolescence, poor diet, and heavy alcohol consumption. Deficiencies in vitamin B12 and C can increase the risk of folate deficiency. Female athletes are at a higher risk of deficiency of folate. Folate deficiency is seen with certain medications, for example, aspirin and oral contraceptives. The body does store small amounts of folic acid in the liver. The RDA for folate is 400 μg/day for males and females. Pregnancy will increase the RDA to 600 μg/day, and lactation will increase the RDA to 500 μg/day. The UL established for folate is 1000 μg/day, and there may be some increase in seizure activity for those taking large doses of folate while using anticonvulsant therapy. Folate may alleviate some of the symptoms of vitamin B12 deficiency, making this harder to diagnose. A lack of folate can have a negative impact on athletic performance. Clinically folate can be used to reduce or prevent congenital disabilities (particularly neural tube defects), reduce atherosclerosis, support depression, improve concentration, support the immune system, and reduce the risk of some cancers. Food sources of folate include animal sources such as calf's liver and eggs and plant sources such as wheat germ, kidney beans, spinach, broccoli, brewer's yeast, and beets [1, 4, 11].

5.4.8 Vitamin B12

The chemical name for vitamin B12 is cobalamin. The body can store small amounts of cobalamin in the liver, decreasing the risk of deficiency. The functions of cobalamin are to assist in the metabolism of folate to THF, the conversion of homocysteine to methionine, fat metabolism, protein synthesis, red blood cell production, nucleic acid synthesis, the synthesis of myelin, and as an antioxidant. A cobalamin deficiency can result in numbness and tingling in the hands and feet, sensory loss, poor coordination and gait, mood changes, memory loss, psychosis, decreased immune response, inflammation of the mucus membranes in the digestive tract, anemia, and reduced platelets. There is an increased risk of deficiency in those who do not eat animal products, those with a decreased production of intrinsic factor which is required for B12 absorption, pregnant and lactating women, those with liver disease, the elderly, those with intestinal disorders, heavy alcohol consumption, and some smoking. Vegetarian athletes are at a higher risk of B12 deficiency. Female athletes are at a higher risk of deficiency of vitamin B12. Some medications may increase the risk of deficiency of cobalamin. The RDA for cobalamin is 2.4 µg/day for both males and females. The RDA increases to 2.6 µg/day during pregnancy and 2.8 µg/day during lactation. No UL is established for cobalamin, and it is generally considered nontoxic. Clinically cobalamin can support some psychiatric conditions, increase energy, reduce atherosclerosis, reduce lung cancer risk, reduce some allergies, and improve some peripheral nerve symptoms and neuropathies. Cobalamin is produced by bacteria, so the food sources of cobalamin are animal in nature, for example, beef, eggs, and salmon. This presents an issue for those who avoid animal products in their diet. This group must be careful to get enough cobalamin, typically through supplementation. The amount of vitamin B12 in food is reduced in the cooking process [1, 4, 11, 12].

5.4.9 Vitamin C

The chemical name for vitamin C is ascorbic acid. The functions of ascorbic acid include antioxidant functions, the synthesis of collagen, the synthesis of carnitine, the production of norepinephrine, epinephrine, and serotonin, support detoxification in the liver, immune support, cholesterol excretion, needed in iron absorption, protects vitamin E and iron, and control histamine levels. Scurvy is a disease associated with vitamin C deficiency. It will show the symptoms of impaired wound healing, easy bruising, bleeding gums, loss of appetite, weakness, fatigue, joint stiffness, and muscle pain. Other signs of deficiency include the thickening of keratin in the skin, depression, and a weakened immune system. An increased risk for deficiency is seen in those who smoke, have increased physical stress, have increased environmental stressors, older individuals, pregnant and lactating women, adolescents, and those who take medications like aspirin and oral contraceptive use. The RDA for vitamin C is 90 mg/day for males and 75 mg/day for females.

The RDA for vitamin C increases to 85 mg/day during pregnancy and 120 mg/day during lactation. There is a UL established for vitamin C at 2000 mg/day. In large doses, some individuals may notice gastrointestinal discomfort and an increased risk of kidney stones. Clinically, vitamin C can be used to support the immune system, reduce the risk of certain cancers, wound healing, reduce atherosclerosis, support asthma, reduce metal toxicity, improve iron absorption from food, support those with diabetes, support periodontal disease, help with hemorrhoids, increase male fertility, and improve glaucoma. Athletes may find that vitamin C administered post-exercise may reduce the impact of exercise-induced oxidated stress. Studies support the increased need for vitamin C for its antioxidant benefits but fall short of recommending supplemental sources, instead suggesting vitamin C comes from the diet. Food sources of vitamin C are primarily from fruit and vegetable sources, including broccoli, citrus fruits, papaya, strawberries, green bell peppers, and potatoes. The content of vitamin C in foods can be reduced when cooking in water, e.g., boiling [1, 4, 13, 14].

5.5 Fat-Soluble Vitamins

5.5.1 Vitamin A

The chemical name for vitamin A is retinol, which can be found in other related forms, such as retinal or retinoic acid. Vitamin A can also be synthesized from precursors in food, referred to as provitamin A. The carotenoids, known for giving foods bright colors, are examples of provitamins. The functions of vitamin A are part of the visual cycle (particularly night vision), stem cell differentiation, maintaining healthy mucus membranes, immune support through lymphocyte generation, support fertility (not retinoic acid), and is essential for bone growth. A deficiency in vitamin A can lead to dryness of the eyes, dry and rough skin with a rash, reduced hormone production, fatigue, poor development, dry, brittle hair and nails, and poor dim light vision. Populations at an increased risk for deficiency include children and adolescents due to rising needs, those experiencing stress, infections and post-surgical due to increased requirements, alcoholism, smokers, those subjected to smoke and or polluted environments, and those with absorption issues with fat. The daily requirements for vitamin A are expressed in retinol activity equivalents or RAE. This accounts for the different potencies of sources, such as retinol vs carotenoids. The RDA for vitamin A is 900 μg RAE/day for males and 700 RAE μ/day for females. The RDA increases to 770 μg RAE/day during pregnancy and 1300 μg RAE/day during lactation.

Vitamin A can be stored in the liver but requires proteins through the bloodstream. A UL is established for vitamin A at 3000 μg RAE/day. Toxicity is associated with the overconsumption of vitamin A or supplementation but not the overconsumption of carotenoids. Toxicity of vitamin A will result in bone pain and joint swelling, dry skin and lips, liver and spleen enlargement, headaches, and blurred vision. During pregnancy, toxicity with vitamin A can be associated with congenital disabilities. Clinically, vitamin A can be used to support the immune system, treat skin and hair issues, improve acne, support wound healing, reduce the symptoms of COPD, support gastric ulcers through increased mucus production, decrease the risk of cataracts, and support iron-deficient anemias. There is evidence that vitamin A may be beneficial in reducing the risk of some cancers. Food sources of vitamin A include beef liver, cod liver oil, eggs, cheese, butter, and milk. Food sources of carotenoids include carrots, sweet potatoes, spinach, apricots, and peaches [1, 4].

5.5.2 Vitamin D

Vitamin D is known by the chemical names cholecalciferol (D3), which comes from foods of animal origin, and ergocalciferol (D2), which comes from food of plant origin. D3 is the preferred source of vitamin D because it has increased bioavailability. Vitamin D from either form can be stored in the liver as 25-OH-vitamin D but must be activated to calcitriol before use. Functionally, calcitriol is more like a hormone and is needed to enhance calcium and phosphorus absorption in the intestine, regulate the calcification of bone tissue, regulate the kidney absorption and excretion of calcium, regulate cellular development in white blood and epithelial cells, and enhance the immune response. Deficiency in vitamin D is associated with rickets in children, symptoms of which include softening of the bones, bowed legs, spinal deformities, swollen joints, and a delay in the closure of the soft spots in the skull. Osteomalacia is a vitamin D deficiency in adults characterized by softening bones, increased risk for osteoporosis and fracture, and hearing loss or ear ringing. Other deficiency symptoms include irritability, restlessness, muscle weakness, increased blood pressure, cancer risk, and impaired immune function. Those at an increased risk of deficiency include those with inadequate sunlight exposure (particularly those living in high latitudes during the winter), the elderly, active individuals who do not get enough dietary vitamin D or sunlight exposure, those whose diets do not contain enough vitamin D, those with fat malabsorption, and those who cannot synthesize vitamin D in the skin. The RDA for vitamin D is 900 IU/day for males and 700 IU/day for females. The RDA increases to 770 IU/day during pregnancy and 1300 IU/day during lactation. The UL for vitamin D is 4000 IU/day. Toxicity may result in hypercalcemia and calcification of soft tissues. Vitamin D toxicity is associated with supplementation and overconsumption rather than too much sun exposure. Clinically, vitamin D can be used for treating bone disorders such as rickets, osteomalacia, and osteoporosis, reduce the severity of psoriasis, enhance immunity and hearing loss, and may be associated with reducing the risk for some cancers. In athletes, vitamin D status is associated with muscle strength, recovery, and fighting off upper respiratory tract infections. Vitamin D has been associated with increasing the number and size of fast-twitch muscle fibers; deficiency can lead to atrophy of these fibers. This has direct implications on speed- and power-based sports. Vitamin D can be found in salmon, tuna, eggs, calf liver, and butter from animal sources. Plant sources of vitamin D are less common but can be found in foods like shitake mushrooms. Vitamin D is also included in food fortification, although this could be in either the D2 or D3 forms. The skin can also synthesize vitamin D3, although the synthesis degree will differ at different latitudes [1, 4, 15, 16].

5.5.3 Vitamin K

Vitamin K refers to a family of three interrelated compounds. Phylloquinone (K1) comes from plant foods, menaquinone (K2) comes from animal sources and is synthesized by the bacteria of the large intestine, and menadione (K3) comes from synthetic sources and is usually used in animal feed. The function of vitamin K is to support blood clotting and as a cofactor in osteocalcin needed to regulate bone metabolism. Deficiency symptoms include increased bleeding before clotting, bruising, blood in the stool, and impaired bone remodeling. Those at an increased risk of deficiency include alcoholics, those with liver disease (the storage site for vitamin K), fat malabsorption, newborns at an increased risk, and those who use some drugs like broad-spectrum antibiotics and blood thinners. The AI for vitamin K is 120 µg/day for males and 90 µg/day for females. No UL is associated with vitamin K, and the forms K1 and K2 are not associated with toxicity. Menadione (K3) can be toxic if ingested in large quantities but is not available in supplements currently. Approximately half of the daily requirements of vitamin K can be met through synthesizing K2 in the large intestine. Clinically vitamin K can treat bleeding disorders in newborns and osteoporosis. Food sources for vitamin K include turnip greens, spinach, broccoli, romaine lettuce, cabbage, soybeans, okra, blackberries, green peas, asparagus, green peas, and artichokes from plants and beef liver, eggs, and butter from animal sources. Vitamin K content can be lost with heat cooking [1, 2].

5.5.4 Vitamin E

Vitamin E refers to a group of eight compounds with similar biological activity. These eight compounds consist of four tocopherols and four tocotrienols. Each is delineated as alpha, beta, gamma, and delta. The most abundant of these is alpha-tocopherol. The different forms of vitamin E have differing bioavailabilities, which must be considered when accounting for daily requirements. Vitamin E is stored in various organs, but the most significant portion is stored in adipose tissue. An essential function of vitamin E is the prevention of oxidation of unsaturated fatty acids, which makes vitamin E a potent antioxidant. As part of its antioxidant role, vitamin E can help to prevent the oxidation of LDL cholesterol, which predisposes the individual to atherosclerotic lesions. Vitamin E also functions to slow down blood clotting without increasing bleeding risk. Symptoms of vitamin E deficiency include skeletal and smooth muscle atrophy and weakness, hemolytic anemia, nerve cell degeneration, atrophy of reproductive organs, and increased risk of cancer, atherosclerosis, arthritis, and cataracts. Those at risk of vitamin E deficiency include newborns, pregnant and lactating women, those with a diet high in polyunsaturated fatty acids, people consuming a poor diet rich in processed foods, those with deficiencies in vitamin C and selenium, those with fat malabsorption, and those who live in environments with high amounts of pollutants and environmental toxins. The RDA for vitamin E is 15 mg/day for males and females. The RDA increases to 19 mg/day for lactating women. A UL of 1000 mg/day has been established for alpha-tocopherol due to the increased risk of bleeding dosages between 200 and 800 mg/day, which may cause some gastrointestinal distress. Clinically, vitamin E can be used to reduce the risk of cardiovascular disease, cataracts, and some cancers, support those with fat malabsorption disorders, support premature infants, benefit those with hemolytic anemia, improve skin conditions, protect from environmental stressors, support premenstrual syndrome, supporting those with Alzheimer's disease, enhanced immune function, support diabetics, and reduce exercise-induced oxidative stress. While vitamin E is a powerful antioxidant that may reduce exercise-induced oxidative stress, supplementation beyond meeting daily requirements is ineffective for athletes. Food sources of vitamin E include plant sources such as plant-based oils, e.g., sunflower and safflower oil, wheat germ, sweet potatoes, shrimp, salmon, and eggs from animal sources. Heat cooking, processing, and storage will reduce the vitamin E availability [1, 4, 14].

5.6 Electrolytes

5.6.1 Sodium

Sodium is the major extracellular (found outside of the cells) cation (positively charged ion) found in the body. Most of the sodium 70% is found in extracellular fluids (such as plasma), nerve, and muscle tissues. The function of sodium is as an electrolyte involved in maintaining osmotic pressure and fluid balance, maintaining the membrane potential of cells, nerve transmission, and muscle contraction. Deficiencies in sodium are rare due to their prevalence in processed foods. Deficiency symptoms include muscle cramps, nausea, vomiting, dizziness, shock, and coma. The AI for sodium is 1500 mg/day for males and females. Over the age of 50, the AI drops to 1300 mg/day and 1200 mg/day over 70 for both males and females. The UL for sodium is 2300 mg/day. Clinically, long-term elevations in sodium are associated with hypertension, increased cancer risk, kidney stones, and osteoporosis. Athletes will require more significant amounts of sodium to account for losses due to sports performance, particularly in warmer weather. In the diet, sodium is primarily found in the form of added salt in the form of sodium chloride or table salt. Processed foods make up much of the sodium in the diet [1, 4, 17].

5.6.2 Chloride

Chloride is an anion (meaning a negatively charged ion) found chiefly in extracellular fluids. The negative charge of chloride will neutralize the positive charge of sodium to create sodium chloride or table salt. It is in the form of sodium chloride that most of the chloride is found in the diet. The function of chloride is as an electrolyte, a component of hydrochloric acid in the stomach for digestion, assisting with immune function, and chloride participates in the chloride shift, which helps remove bicarbonate from the blood. A deficiency in chloride is not seen during normal physiological function. Deficiencies are associated with gastrointestinal issues such as severe diarrhea or vomiting. The AI for chloride is 2300 mg/day for males and females. Over the age of 50, the AI drops to 2000 mg/day and 1800 mg/day over 70 for both males and females. The UL for chloride is 3600 mg/day. Athletes will require more significant amounts of chloride to account for losses due to sports performance. Food sources of chloride are associated primarily with added salt in the diet, which is the most abundant form of chloride. Chloride is also found in eggs, fresh meats, and seafood [1, 4, 17].

5.6.3 Potassium

Most of the potassium is contained intracellularly (or within the cells). Potassium's functions are essential for energy metabolism, membrane excitability, and transport, e.g., muscle contraction and nerve transmission. Signs of deficiency include low blood pressure, muscle weakness, cardiac arrhythmias, delayed gastric emptying, constipation, and fatigue. The risk of potassium deficiency is increased with diarrhea, vomiting, chronic kidney failure, extreme long-term dieting, alterations in body pH, many diuretics, and those with deficiency. The AI for potassium is 4700 mg/day for males and females. The AI increases to 5100 mg/day for lactating women. Clinically, potassium can treat high blood pressure, replace potassium lost with diarrhea and cardiac arrhythmias, and support athletes by replacing potassium lost in sweat. Food sources of potassium include soy, white beans, lentils, bananas, spinach, whole wheat bread, rye bread, potatoes, orange juice, vegetables, and almonds from plant sources and fish, beef, and chicken from animal sources [1, 4, 17].

5.7 Major Minerals

5.7.1 Calcium

Calcium is the most abundant mineral in the body. Most of the calcium in the body is found in the bones and teeth. Calcium gives the bones and teeth structure, supports the blood clotting cascade, and triggers muscle contractions and nerve transmission. Calcium deficiencies lead to osteoporosis, poor dental enamel, muscle cramping and spasm, increased nerve irritability, and poor blood clotting. Those at risk for deficiency include menopausal women, atrophic gastritis, inadequate dietary intake, vitamin D deficiency, malabsorption syndromes, and medications like laxatives, antacids, and steroids. Female athletes are at a higher risk of calcium deficiency if dairy and calcium-containing foods are not abundant in their diet. The RDA for calcium is 1000 mg/day for males and females, increasing to 1200 mg/day for females over 50 and males over 70. The UL for calcium is 2500 mg/day between the ages of 19 and 50 and 2000 mg/day over 50. The UL is 2500 mg/day during pregnancy and lactation. Clinically, calcium is essential for reducing the risk of colon cancer, high blood pressure, osteoporosis, periodontal disease, and lead toxicity and supporting those with digestive disorders like Crohn's and celiac disease. Calcium absorption and retention may be reduced with diets high in protein (>20% of daily calories), oxalates, phytic acid, sodium, alcohol, coffee, and black tea. Calcium may help to reduce the risk of exercise-related stress fractures in athletes. Calcium is also essential for muscle contractions and deficiencies associated with cramping. Calcium food sources include kale, broccoli, cabbage, fennel, cauliflower, oranges, and soybeans from plant sources and milk, cheese, yogurt, and sardines from animal sources. Calcium bioavailability is less for plant sources due to oxalates and phytic acid [1, 4, 17, 18].

5.7.2 Phosphorus

Phosphorus is the second most abundant mineral in the body. Functionally, phosphorus is essential in bone mineralization (85% of phosphorus is found in the skeleton), plays a role in enzyme activity, is a component of cell membranes, plays a role in acid-base balance, and phosphorus is an essential component of nucleic acids, ATP/ADP, cAMP, and creatine phosphate. Deficiency is rare, often seed with significant antacid use and refeeding syndrome. Deficiency symptoms include anorexia, leukocyte dysfunction, reduced cardiac output, arrhythmias, and skeletal and cardiac myopathy. The RDA for phosphorus is 700 mg/day for males and females. The UL for phosphorus is 4000 mg/day between 19 and 70 and 3000 mg/day over 70. The UL is 3500 mg/day during pregnancy and 4000 mg/day during lactation. Toxicity, while rare, can result in tetany and calcification of tissues (particularly the kidneys). Food sources of phosphorus include meat, poultry, fish, eggs, and milk from animal sources and nuts, legumes, grains, and cereals from plant sources. Typically, animal sources of phosphorus are more bioavailable [1, 4, 17].

5.7.3 Magnesium

Magnesium is an abundant mineral in the human body. Sixty percent of magnesium is stored in the skeletal tissue. Magnesium has essential functions in energy production, cardiac and skeletal muscle contractions, hormonal function, stimulating vasodilation in blood vessels, regulating nerve depolarization, and supporting the structure of bones and teeth. A magnesium deficiency can result in muscle cramps and spasms, impaired insulin secretion, depression, irritability, anorexia, nausea, vomiting, arrhythmias, insufficient action of vitamin D, increased cholesterol and triglycerides, a potential increase in calcium and potassium losses, and sodium and water retention. Populations at an increased risk for deficiency include athletes, children and adolescents, pregnancy, lactation, diabetics, alcoholics, those with malabsorption syndromes, and some medications such as diuretics and chemotherapy. The RDA for magnesium is 400 mg/day for males between 19 and 30 and 420 mg/day over 30. The RDA for females is 310 mg/day between 19 and 30 and 320 mg/day over the age of 30. The RDA is 700 mg/day during pregnancy and lactation. The UL for magnesium is 350 mg/day. Signs of toxicity include nausea, flushing, weakness, double vision, and slurred speech. Clinically, magnesium is used to prevent seizures with preeclampsia/eclampsia, hypertension, cardiovascular disease, diabetes, migraines, anxiety, insomnia, muscle cramps, osteoporosis, and premenstrual syndrome. In athletes, magnesium deficiency can reduce endurance performance. Magnesium is associated with muscle cramping. Magnesium deficiency is more common in athletes who compete in weight-dependent sports, where an athlete may need to rapidly lose weight before competition. Food sources of magnesium include soy flour, whole rice, barley, wheat bran, sunflower seeds, whole wheat bread, lentils, wheat germ, walnuts, peanuts, almonds, and spinach [1, 4, 17].

5.8 Essential Trace Minerals

5.8.1 Iron

Iron is an essential mineral found in various forms in the body. The Fe^{3+} ferric and Fe^{2+} ferrous forms are the most important. Iron can be stored in the body's tissues, with men typically storing approx. 3.8 g and women storing approx. 2.3 g. The functions of iron include oxygen delivery as part of hemoglobin in blood and storage as myoglobin in muscle, energy production, gene regulation, cell growth, and differentiation, and as a cofactor in several enzyme systems such as cytochrome p450. Symptoms of iron deficiency include anemia, fatigue, loss of appetite, inability to maintain warmth, difficulties with learning, memory, and concentration, impaired mental and motor development in children, inflammation of the oral mucosa, increased risk of infection, increased risk of lead and cadmium intake, and in athletes decreased performance. Populations at risk of deficiency include women, those undergoing rapid growth such as childhood and adolescents, pregnancy, vegetarians and other diets low in iron, reduced gastric secretions, those with heavy menstruation, endurance athletes, those with deficiencies in vitamin A, B6, and copper. The RDA for iron is 8 mg/day for males and 18 mg/day for females between 19 and 50, and 8 mg/day for females over 50. The RDA increases to 27 mg/day during pregnancy and 9 mg/day during lactation. The UL for iron is 45 mg/day. The symptoms of toxicity include gastrointestinal discomfort, such as abdominal pain, nausea, and vomiting. Iron toxicity can be fatal in children and those with hemochromatosis. Toxicity is more common with supplementation than with whole foods. Clinically iron is associated with treating iron-deficient anemias, fatigue, low energy, learning difficulties, some infections, and supporting pregnancy. Athletes who compete in endurance sports will benefit from ensuring they have accounted for their increased needs. Sustained bouts of exercise can be associated with increases in hepcidin. This hormone regulates iron homeostasis, which can lead to reductions in iron stores, supporting the higher rates of iron deficiency in athletes. Female athletes are at a higher risk for deficiency than males due to losses seen with menstruation. Evaluation and early treatment of reduced iron in athletes can improve work capacity and endurance, increase oxygen uptake, reduce lactic acid conversion, and reduce muscle fatigue. Food sources of iron include beef and pork liver, oysters, beef, pork, chicken, and eggs from animal sources and soy flour, lentils, white beans, oatmeal, rye, whole rice, dried figs, dried apricots, whole wheat bread, carrots, zucchini, and dried dates from plant sources. Animal sources have a higher bioavailability of iron compared to plant sources. Oral supplementation should consider the ferrous form that may help reduce gastrointestinal distress [1, 4, 17–19].

5.8.2 Zinc

Zinc is a trace element that is widely distributed in the body. The wide distribution of zinc relates to the numerous functions ranging from gene expression to immune function. Zinc is required to support the function of more than 200 enzymes impacting both structure and activity. Zinc plays a vital role in the structure and function of proteins, energy production, gene expression, immune function, antioxidant functions, the release of certain hormones, and protection from some toxic compounds. A zinc deficiency will result in dermatitis, reduced smell and taste, reduced vitamin A metabolism, slowed growth, delayed sexual maturity, depression, irritability, fatigue, poor concentration, weakened immunity, and unusual cravings such as dirt. Populations at an increased risk for deficiency include children, adolescents, pregnant and lactating women, those on long-term diets, vegetarians, those with malabsorption syndromes, those taking high-dose calcium supplements, alcoholics, diabetics, and those with liver or kidney diseases. The RDA for zinc is 11 mg/day for males and 8 mg/day for females. The RDA increases to 11 mg/day during pregnancy and 12 mg/day during lactation. The UL for zinc is 40 mg/day. Zinc toxicity may result in nausea, vomiting, bloody diarrhea, abdominal cramps, weakness, sweating, and copper deficiency. Clinically, zinc is used to prevent and treat macular degeneration, support wound healing, enhance immunity, support growth and development, improve male fertility, support some skin conditions, and help support those with inflammatory arthritis. Female athletes are at a higher risk of deficiency of zinc. In athletes, decreased zinc has been associated with lower cardiorespiratory function, muscle strength, and endurance. Zinc supplementation can lead to excesses that can impair the absorption of other minerals, such as iron and copper, impacting performance. Food sources of zinc include calf liver, oysters, beef, chicken, seafood, and eggs from animal sources, as well as lentils, green peas, whole wheat bread, wheat bran, corn, and oatmeal from plant sources. Animal sources of zinc are more bioavailable than plant sources, which is why vegetarians are at a greater risk of deficiency. Cooking will decrease the bioavailability of zinc [1, 4, 18].

5.8.3 Iodine

Iodine is a widespread mineral deficiency in countries outside of the United States. The deficiency is mitigated in the United States due to using iodized table salt. Table salt does bring other health issues, but as far as iodine is concerned, it does decrease deficiency. The functions of iodine are involved in the synthesis of thyroid hormones. Signs of iodine deficiency include goiter, hypothyroidism, impaired mental function, cretinism in children and infants, increased infant mortality, abortions, stillbirths, congenital disabilities, and impaired physical growth. Populations at an increased risk of deficiency are those that live far from the coast, particularly where soil may be depleted of iodine, pregnant and lactating women, diets low in iodine or rich in foods that block the uptake of iodine, such as cassava and sweet potatoes. The RDA for iodine is 150 µg/day for males and females. The RDA increases to 220 µg/day during pregnancy and 290 µg/day during lactation. The UL for iodine is 1100 µg/day. Toxicity can result in nausea, vomiting, burning in the throat and mouth, diarrhea, and fever. Clinically, iodine can be associated with iodine-caused hypothyroidism and supports the diets of those at risk for deficiency. Food sources of iodine include mussels, clams, salmon, shrimp, cod, mackerel, tuna, herring, and halibut. Iodized salt is also a significant source of iodine in the standard diet [1, 4].

5.8.4 Selenium

Selenium is a nonmetal element found in all human tissues. Selenium functions as an antioxidant, supports immune function, has a role in pancreatic function, aids in DNA repair, and is required to convert T4 to T3 in the thyroid. A selenium deficiency will present with decreased resistance to oxidative damage, a form of childhood osteoarthritis called Kashin–Beck disease, muscle weakness, cardiomyopathy, heart failure (Keshan disease), increased risk of infection, and increased cancer risk. The populations with an increased risk of deficiency include those needing increased selenium due to increased oxidative load, including smokers, strenuous exercisers, and those exposed to oxidative stress. Additionally, those on para-enteral nutrition, those with malabsorption issues, and those living in areas with low selenium content in the soil may have an increased risk of deficiency. The RDA for selenium is 55 µg/day for males and females. The RDA increases to 60 µg/day during pregnancy and 70 µg/day during lactation. The UL for selenium is 400 µg/day. Toxicity from selenium can result in nausea, vomiting, diarrhea, hair loss, fatigue, and peripheral neuropathy. Clinically, selenium is used to help lower the risk for some cancers like lung, colon, and prostate. Selenium can support chronic inflammatory diseases, those with infectious diseases, heart disease patients, and some patients with hypothyroidism, help with Kashin–Beck arthritis, and limit the accumulation of heavy metals from food and water. Selenium as an antioxidant is important to limit the effects of exercise-induced oxidative damage. Food sources of selenium include tuna, herring, sardines, calf liver, beef, pork, salmon, cod, and milk from animal products and soybeans, white beans, whole wheat bread, and certain nuts like Brazil nuts. The content of selenium in food will vary based on the content of selenium in the soil [1, 4, 14, 18].

5.8.5 Copper

The functions of copper in the body include energy production, the metabolism of iron, connective tissue synthesis and wound healing, as an antioxidant, synthesis of melanin, and the metabolism of hormones and neurotransmitters. Signs of a copper deficiency include anemia, abnormal skeletal growth, osteoporosis, hair loss, pigment loss, vitiligo, weakness, fatigue, increased cholesterol, triglycerides, glucose intolerance, aneurism risk, and decreased immune response. Populations at an increased risk of deficiency include high intakes of iron, molybdenum, or zinc; infants fed only cows' milk. Prolonged antacid use – gastrointestinal disorders that decrease absorption, smoking, and increased environmental stressors. The RDA for copper is 900 μg/day for males and females. The RDA increases to 1000 μg/day during pregnancy and 1300 μg/day during lactation. The UL for copper is 10 000 μg/day. Toxicity can be associated with abdominal pain, nausea, vomiting, diarrhea, and liver damage. Wilson's disease is genetic, resulting in decreased copper excretion and toxic buildup. Clinically, copper can be used to treat anemia (if caused by copper deficiency), rheumatoid arthritis, and cardiovascular disease, improve immune function, and support those taking large doses of zinc. Food sources of copper include calf liver, oysters, hard cheeses, chicken beef, and chicken from animal sources and lentils, chickpeas, kidney beans, sunflower seeds, hazelnuts, walnuts, almonds, dried apricots, and some port wines, and sherry from plant sources [1, 4, 14].

5.8.6 Manganese

Manganese functions in the body to support carbohydrate metabolism, support insulin production, as an antioxidant, support protein metabolism, support bone and cartilage synthesis, and the activation of enzymes necessary for various activities. The signs and symptoms of a manganese deficiency include reduced HDL cholesterol, increased liver fat, glucose intolerance due to decreased insulin secretion, decreased appetite, weight loss, impaired bone production, dermatitis, reduced hair, and nail growth, and increased susceptibility to oxidative damage. The populations at risk of deficiency include those with low dietary intake from diets high in processed foods, refined carbohydrates, and rich in animal products, those exposed to increased environmental pollutants that would increase oxidant production, alcoholics, smokers, and high iron intake. The AI for manganese is 2.3 mg/day for males and 1.8 mg/day for females. The AI increases to 2.0 mg/day during pregnancy and 2.6 mg/day during lactation. The UL for manganese is 11 mg/day. Toxicity of manganese can result in psychosis, hyperirritability, violent behavior, lack of coordination, dementia, and symptoms similar to Parkinson's disease. Clinically, manganese can be used to treat osteoporosis, diabetes, epilepsy, asthma, and premenstrual syndrome. Food sources of manganese include oatmeal, soy flour, whole wheat flour, hazelnuts, whole wheat bread, wheat germ, white beans, dried apricots, dried figs, walnuts, almonds, whole rice, black tea, and coffee. Dietary intake of iron and phytates can reduce manganese absorption [1, 4, 14, 19].

5.8.7 Chromium

Chromium is an essential trace element. The function of chromium is for carbohydrate metabolism by improving glucose tolerance, supporting lipid metabolism, supporting protein metabolism, and enhancing RNA synthesis. Signs of chromium deficiency include reduced glucose tolerance, weight loss, elevated cholesterol and triglycerides, and peripheral neuropathy. Populations at increased risk of deficiency include diets low in chromium and high in refined grains, those with increased physical stress due to exercise, physical activity, infection, trauma, or illness, pregnant women, and the elderly. The AI for chromium is 35 µg/day for males between the ages of 19 and 50 and 30 µg/day over 50. The AI for females is 25 µg/day between the ages of 19 and 50 and 20 µg/day over 50. The AI increases to 30 µg/day during pregnancy and 45 µg/day during lactation. Clinically chromium can support glucose tolerance, as seen in type 2 diabetes, supporting lipid biomarkers by lowering LDL, total cholesterol, and triglycerides and raising HDL cholesterol, supporting recovery from physical stressors such as exercise, trauma, surgery, and illness. Chromium food sources include lentils, whole wheat bread, molasses, and Brewer's yeast from plant sources and chicken from animal sources. Ascorbic acid or vitamin C increases the absorption of chromium [1, 4, 20].

5.8.8 Molybdenum

Molybdenum is an essential trace mineral. Functionally molybdenum is an antioxidant that supports the detoxification and excretion of chemicals and drugs, iron metabolism, and sulfur metabolism. The signs of a molybdenum deficiency include decreased antioxidant protection, impaired sulfur metabolism, increased sensitivity of sulfites, hair loss, fatigue, increased risk of esophageal cancer, and increased risk of kidney stones. Populations at risk for deficiency include diets rich in refined carbohydrates, fats, oils, and meat products, chronic exposure to drugs and chemicals, and digestive disorders that lead to increased molybdenum loss, such as diarrhea. The RDA for molybdenum is 45 µg/day for males and females. The RDA increases to 50 µg/day during pregnancy and lactation. The UL for molybdenum is 2000 µg/day. The toxicity of molybdenum can lead to increased uric acid production and gout. Clinically, molybdenum can reduce sulfite sensitivity, mitigate toxicity from foreign substances like drugs and chemicals, and reduce the risk of some cancers. Food sources of molybdenum include soy flour, red cabbage, white beans, potatoes, whole rice, green peas, spinach, green beans, whole wheat bread, and wheat germ from plant sources and eggs from animal sources [1, 4].

5.9 Nonessential Trace Minerals and Choline

5.9.1 Fluoride

Fluoride is a nutrient once considered essential but is now classified as beneficial. The benefits of fluoride are the direct relationship between fluoride and reduced dental caries. The functions of fluoride are to support tooth structure and stimulate osteoblast activity, supporting bone production. The signs and symptoms of fluoride deficiency are an increased risk of dental caries. The AI for fluoride is 4 mg/day for males and 3 mg/day for females. The UL for fluoride is 10 mg/day. Fluoride toxicity can result in dental fluorosis, skeletal deformities, osteoporosis, osteomalacia, secondary hyperparathyroidism, and calcification of soft tissues. Clinically, fluoride is used for prophylactic dental caries protection and to treat osteoporosis. Food sources of fluoride include canned sardines, tea, and fluoridated salt chicken. Fluoridated water is also a significant source of fluoride [1, 4].

5.9.2 Arsenic

Arsenic is a nonessential trace element that facilitates the use of methyl groups, regulates signal transduction, and influences cell proliferation and survival. A deficiency in arsenic can result in impaired metabolism of methionine, diminished growth, reduced conception rate, abnormal reproduction, increased neonatal mortality, and altered lipid concentrations. Although some evidence supports 12–25 µg/day, no RDA or AI has been established for arsenic. There has been no UL established for arsenic. Despite lacking an UL, arsenic, acute toxicity can result in gastrointestinal distress, encephalopathy, anemia, and liver damage. Chronic toxicity can result in skin hyperpigmentation, hyperkeratosis, muscle weakness, peripheral neuropathy, sweating, liver damage, delirium, encephalopathy, vascular changes, increased risk of some cancers, hypertension, and arrhythmias. Clinically, arsenic has been used to treat leukemia. Food sources for arsenic include fish, oysters, meats, eggs, and milk from animal sources and cereal and grains from plant sources [1, 4].

5.9.3 Boron

Boron is a nonessential trace element that is used, in various forms, as a preserving agent in foods. Functionally, boron is shown to have effects on bones, cell membranes, the immune system, and the brain, although specific functions have been identified. Decreased levels of boron are associated with decreased cytokines, antibodies, white blood cells, impaired memory, reduced attention span, and impaired growth and development. There is no established RDA or AI for boron, but intakes of 1–3 mg/day are suggested as beneficial. A UI of 20 mg/day of boron has been established with acute toxicity resulting in nausea, vomiting, diarrhea, dermatitis, and lethargy. Chronic toxicity is associated with nausea, poor appetite, anemia, dermatitis, and seizures. Food sources of boron include meat, fish, and dairy from animal sources and avocados, peanuts, peanut butter, pecans, raisins, grapes, and wine from plant sources [1, 4].

5.9.4 Nickel

Nickel is a nonessential trace mineral associated with methionine metabolism; nickel can substitute for other minerals, such as magnesium or zinc, in some enzymes, making the enzyme more stable and active. Despite the roles stated, nickel has no defined functions in the body. A deficiency in nickel can result in decreased reproduction and growth and altered iron, lipid, carbohydrate, bone, and thyroid metabolism. No RDA is established for nickel, but the estimated need is less than 100 µg/day. The UL for nickel is 1.0 mg/day. Acute toxicity will result in headaches, nausea, vomiting, insomnia, and irritability. Symptoms can progress to include chest tightness, cough, difficulty breathing, tachycardia, palpitations, sweating, weakness, and death. Chronic toxicity will result in respiratory disorders and an increased risk for some cancers. Nickel food sources include nuts, legumes, grains, and chocolate from plants, fish, milk, and animal eggs. Plant sources contain higher nickel content compared to animal sources [1, 4].

5.9.5 Silicon

Silicon is a nonessential trace mineral found in abundance on the planet. The functions of silicon include bone, cartilage, and connective tissue formation and development. Deficiencies in silicon can result in alterations in bone formation, particularly the long bones and skull. No RDA has been established for silicon, but the estimated requirement for silicon is 10–25 mg/day. No UL has been established for silicon, although 1750 mg/day has been suggested. The toxicity of silicon has been associated with kidney stones, decreased action of some enzymes, increased risk of free radical damage, and respiratory disorders. Food sources of silicon include whole grains and root vegetables. Silicon is also present in water [1, 4].

5.9.6 Vanadium

Vanadium is a nonessential trace mineral with functions associated with bone and energy formation and antioxidant effects. Deficiencies in vanadium are associated with survival, growth, and development decreases. No RDA is established for vanadium, but 10 μg/day has been suggested as required. An UL of 1.8 mg/day has been established. Toxicity can result in discoloration of the tongue (green tongue syndrome), diarrhea, gastrointestinal cramping, hypertension, neurological disorders, and hepatic, cardiac, and renal damage. Clinically, vanadium has been associated with cardiovascular support following a heart attack and support for those with type 2 diabetes. Vanadium food sources include black pepper, parsley, dill seed, canned apple juice, fish sticks, mushrooms, cereals, grains, beer, and wine from plant sources [1, 4].

5.9.7 Choline

Choline is an essential element needed to produce cell membranes. The functions of choline include the formation of cell membranes, the formation of myelin, the synthesis of the neurotransmitter acetylcholine, and the metabolism of fats and triglycerides in the liver. Symptoms of choline deficiency include fat accumulation in the liver, impaired kidney function, decreased hematopoiesis, hypertension, abnormal growth, difficulty with learning and memory, reduced carnitine metabolism, and an increased risk of liver cancer. Populations at risk of choline deficiency are alcoholics, diets low in folate, those with poor absorptions such as pancreatic or intestinal diseases, and those with AIDS. The AI for choline is 550 mg/day for males and 425 mg/day for females. The AI increases to 450 mg/day during pregnancy and 550 mg/day during lactation. The UL for choline is 3500 mg/day. Choline toxicity has been associated with nausea, vomiting, depression, dizziness, and body odor. Clinically, choline has been associated with improved lipid biomarkers, improved memory, supporting Alzheimer's patients, support for some mental health conditions, pregnancy support, support for heavy alcohol consumption, reduced symptoms and duration of hepatitis, and reduced incidence of gallstones. Choline can improve the performance of endurance athletes. Food sources of choline include calf liver, eggs, and beef from animal sources and peanuts, cauliflower, iceberg lettuce, and whole wheat bread from plant sources [1, 4, 21].

5.10 Conclusion

Dietary macronutrients are crucial to both the health and the performance of athletes. Many of the aforementioned macronutrients have a direct impact on the body's ability to generate energy, produce blood cells, recover from exercise, and have a healthy immune response. A deficiency in any of these micronutrients will negatively impact athletic performance through impairment in the aforementioned processes. In many cases, the need for micronutrients will increase for older athletes, making the requirements to prevent deficiency higher. Although micronutrient deficiencies are rare, a well-rounded diet that is rich in micronutrients will assist the nutritional practitioner in ensuring the nutrients needed from the diet. In this regard, I would suggest that the nutritional practitioner have the athlete complete a food diary so that they will log nutrient intake. The data can be put into one of many computer programs, if the food diary is not kept on a computer database already. These programs analyze many of the aforementioned micronutrients, while this may not be a perfect assessment of micronutrient status, this can tell the provider which micronutrients may be deficient and need to be increased. Much of the research on these nutrients support their needs for athletic performance, but few vitamins show a performance benefit beyond the daily requirements, meaning that once the athlete is getting their needs met, more of the nutrient will not help (Figure 5.7). Others, like vitamin D, do show some performance benefits indicating some benefit from supplementation, to be discussed in Chapter 10.

Energy production			Tissue repair		Antioxidants	
Thiamine	Pyridoxine	Iron	Folate*		Vitamin C	Iron
Riboflavin	Pantothenic acid	Copper	Vitamin B12*		Vitamin E	Zinc
Niacin	Biotin	Chromium			Vitamin A	Copper
Zinc	Magnesium		**Bone support**		Selenium	
			Vitamin D	Magnesium		
Protein synthesis			Calcium		**Blood clotting**	
Folate	Magnesium				Calcium	
Vitamin B 12	Zinc					
Iron					**Red blood cell/Hemoglobin production***	
					Folate	Pyridoxine
Nerve function and muscle contraction			**Immune support**		Vitamin B 12*	Iron
Thaimin	Pyridoxine		Pyridoxine*	Vitamin C	**Membrane stability***	
Riboflavin*	Folic Acid		Vitamin A	Vitamin E*	Magnesium	
Niacin*	Vitamin B12		Vitamin D	Magnesium*		
Sodium	Calcium		Zinc		**Hormonal support***	
Potassium	Magnesium				Magnesium	

Figure 5.7 Micronutrients directly associated with athletic performance [20].

References

1. Gropper SS, Smith JL. *Advanced Nutrition and Human Metabolism*. Cengage Learning, 2018.
2. Institute of Medicine (US) Standing Committee on the Scientific Evaluation of Dietary Reference Intakes. Dietary reference intakes. Dietary Reference Intakes for Calcium, Phosphorus, Magnesium, Vitamin D, and Fluoride, 1997.
3. Institute of Medicine (US) Committee to Review Dietary Reference Intakes for Vitamin D and Calcium. Ross AC, Taylor CL, Yaktine AL, Del Valle HB, eds. *Dietary Reference Intakes for Calcium and Vitamin D*. Washington (DC): National Academies Press (US), 2011.
4. Zimmerman M. *Burgerstein's Handbook of Nutrition: Micronutrients in the Prevention and Therapy of Disease*. Thieme, 2001.
5. Hrubša M, Siatka T, Nejmanová I, et al. Biological properties of vitamins of the B-complex, Part 1: vitamins B_1, B_2, B_3, and B_5. *Nutrients* 2022;14(3):484. Published 2022 Jan 22. doi:10.3390/nu14030484
6. Nichols QZ, Ramadoss R, Stanzione JR, Volpe SL. Micronutrient supplement intakes among collegiate and masters athletes: a cross-sectional study. *Front. Sports Act. Living* 2023;5:854442. Published 2023 Apr 6. doi:10.3389/fspor.2023.854442
7. Lieberman HR, Agarwal S, Fulgoni VL 3rd. Tryptophan intake in the US adult population is not related to liver or kidney function but is associated with depression and sleep outcomes. *J. Nutr.* 2016;146(12):2609S–2615S. doi:10.3945/jn.115.226969
8. Webster MJ. Physiological and performance responses to supplementation with thiamin and pantothenic acid derivatives. *Eur. J. Appl. Physiol. Occup. Physiol.* 1998;77(6):486–491. doi:10.1007/s004210050364
9. Manore MM. Vitamin B6 and exercise. *Int. J. Sport Nutr.* 1994;4(2):89–103. doi:10.1123/ijsn.4.2.89
10. Manore MM. Effect of physical activity on thiamine, riboflavin, and vitamin B-6 requirements. *Am. J. Clin. Nutr.* 2000;72(2 Suppl):598S–606S. doi:10.1093/ajcn/72.2.598S
11. Lukaski HC. Vitamin and mineral status: effects on physical performance. *Nutrition.* 2004;20(7–8):632–644. doi:10.1016/j.nut.2004.04.001
12. West S, Monteyne AJ, van der Heijden I, Stephens FB, Wall BT. Nutritional considerations for the vegan athlete. *Adv. Nutr.* 2023;14(4):774–795. doi:10.1016/j.advnut.2023.04.012
13. Rogers DR, Lawlor DJ, Moeller JL. Vitamin C supplementation and athletic performance: a review. *Curr. Sports Med. Rep.* 2023;22(7):255–259. Published 2023 Jul 1. doi:10.1249/JSR.0000000000001083

14 Higgins MR, Izadi A, Kaviani M. Antioxidants and exercise performance: with a focus on vitamin E and C supplementation. *Int. J. Environ. Res. Public Health* 2020;17(22):8452. Published 2020 Nov 15. doi:10.3390/ijerph17228452

15 Książek A, Zagrodna A, Słowińska-Lisowska M. Vitamin D, Skeletal muscle function and athletic performance in athletes – a narrative review. *Nutrients* 2019;11(8):1800. Published 2019 Aug 4. doi:10.3390/nu11081800

16 Knechtle B, Nikolaidis PT. Vitamin D and sport performance. *Nutrients* 2020;12(3):841. Published 2020 Mar 21. doi:10.3390/nu12030841

17 Orrù S, Imperlini E, Nigro E, et al. Role of functional beverages on sport performance and recovery. *Nutrients* 2018;10(10):1470. Published 2018 Oct 10. doi:10.3390/nu10101470

18 van Dronkelaar C, van Velzen A, Abdelrazek M, et al. Minerals and sarcopenia; the role of calcium, iron, magnesium, phosphorus, potassium, selenium, sodium, and zinc on muscle mass, muscle strength, and physical performance in older adults: a systematic review. *J. Am. Med. Dir. Assoc.* 2018;19(1):6–11.e3. doi:10.1016/j.jamda.2017.05.026

19 Heffernan SM, Horner K, De Vito G, Conway GE. The role of mineral and trace element supplementation in exercise and athletic performance: a systematic review. *Nutrients* 2019;11(3):696. Published 2019 Mar 24. doi:10.3390/nu11030696

20 Lefavi RG, Anderson RA, Keith RE, et al. Efficacy of chromium supplementation in athletes: emphasis on anabolism. *Int. J. Sport Nutr.* 1992;2(2):111–122. doi:10.1123/ijsn.2.2.111

21 Penry JT, Manore MM. Choline: an important micronutrient for maximal endurance-exercise performance?*Int. J. Sport Nutr. Exerc. Metab.* 2008;18(2):191–203. doi:10.1123/ijsnem.18.2.191

6

Nutrition Assessment

6.1 Introduction

A very important element that must be considered when creating a targeted nutritional strategy is the assessment of the current state of the athlete's diet and physical presentation. Although in many cases, a nutritional practitioner will be planning on making a lot of changes in what the athlete is eating as part of their strategy, a look at the current nutritional and physical state of the athlete may provide some insight as to how the athlete functions under current nutritional plans. A client history, assessment of their current diet, anthropometric testing, body composition testing, and any available laboratory information all assist the nutritional practitioner in being able to design a nutritional plan that will best suit the needs of the athlete to achieve their goals. This chapter will discuss many of the common nutritional assessment tools used by a sports nutritionist as well as some general assessment tools that are commonly used.

6.2 Client History

Although not a direct measurement of the athlete's nutrition, a good client history will be an invaluable tool for the nutritional practitioner to use in the determination of the athlete's needs. A history is the first thing done by any practitioner when working with a client or patient. In the case of someone with a medical condition, the history involves questioning the individual about why they are in the office and what their signs and symptoms are. In this case, the athlete will be questioned about why they are in the office and what they hope to achieve from working with the nutritional practitioner. This should be done before assessing the athlete's current nutritional status.

Sports Nutrition for Masters Athletes, First Edition. Peter G. Nickless.
© 2025 John Wiley & Sons, Inc. Published 2025 by John Wiley & Sons, Inc.

To perform a history in this context, the athlete should first be asked questions about their sport. They should describe what training and competition are like including the number of training sessions and duration, frequency and duration of competition, and the perceived intensity of both training and competition. The athlete should then be asked to provide any data they can regarding their current personal bests in their sport; this can be a single metric or several metrics. Following this, the athlete should be asked about their performance and any aesthetic goals both long term and short term. This information is useful in guiding the nutritional suggestions toward assisting the athlete to achieve their goals. The athlete should be asked about any previous sports nutritional work, either done by themselves or another practitioner. This will give an idea of what has been tried, and what has and has not worked. If there have been previous attempts with nutrition, ask about compliance and success, and if there was no success why this was the case. The athlete should be asked about any relevant personal or family medical history. Although the nutritional provider is not looking to treat any specific condition, this information may help the practitioner know of any concerns that may impact the nutritional plan. The final question you should ask the athlete is if there is anything else about themselves that they would like to share. This open-ended question may be useless or may provide the opening for the athlete to indicate a key piece of information needed to determine their nutritional strategy.

6.3 Dietary Analysis

In order to properly address the nutritional needs of an athlete, it is essential that the nutritional provider can assess the current eating habits of the athletes they are working with. The benefits of dietary assessment are that it allows for the evaluation of current dietary habits to help identify any areas of deficiency or excesses in consumption. Additionally, it may help to provide some insight into preferences of the athlete. This information may be helpful in identifying the food types that an athlete enjoys. If an athlete notes that they eat a lot of convenience foods, for example, we may use this information to make appropriate performance-based suggestions that may also be convenient. On the other hand, this may provide insights as to foods that you should consider avoiding with the athlete. If, for example, the athlete reports that they traditionally avoid fish, then the nutritional plan may want to avoid fish. It is therefore important that anyone working with athletes should evaluate the current diet of any athlete they are working with. There are a variety of dietary assessment options available to use. Some of these are snapshots of a single period in time, like a 24-hour food recall, while others are more like looking at the average consumption of foods, as is the case for a food frequency questionnaire. Each dietary assessment has some benefits and drawbacks. In this section, we will explore dietary assessment techniques.

6.3.1 24-Hour Food Recall

The first dietary assessment method we will examine is a simple 24-hour food recall. This is a basic assessment that can be done at any time by anyone. The athlete is simply asked to write down exactly what they ate over the past 24 hours including approximate amounts, times, preparation methods, and brands if known. This food recall can be done during, or prior to, an initial evaluation with an athlete, as well as at all subsequent follow-up visits as a means of assessing compliance to the nutritional plan. The key benefit is that the evaluator gets a one-day snapshot into the dietary life of an athlete. This is not an estimate or a generalization of eating habits, but rather a list of foods that have actually been eaten. This of course is also a drawback as many of us have days that are not always representative of our true dietary patterns. Most people would hate to think that a diet recall taken the day after Thanksgiving could be used as a proxy for their entire diet. This type of recall gives us a great idea of what someone has eaten but not always how often they eat these items. One modification could be to extend the time that the athlete is asked to recall their diet; while this would paint a more complete picture of the diet it may also be difficult to remember longer periods of time. Another drawback to the use of the 24-hour food recall is that it should not be used as an assessment of micronutrients as not all nutrients can and would be consumed in a specific day. Follow-up reevaluations with an athlete should consider using a 24-hour recall, unless some other more ongoing assessment is used like a food dairy, as it can give an indication of compliance and understanding of food recommendations. A simple misunderstanding of instructions can be illuminated easily by examining just what someone ate in the past 24 hours. If I am suggesting meals with a total protein intake of 40 g each and one is consuming a 20 oz steak, which would contain 140 g of protein, then further investigation would be required. In this manner, a 24-hour food recall is a useful nutritional assessment tool for initial and ongoing use.

6.3.2 Food Diaries

When a nutritional practitioner is trying to get the most accurate assessment of the dietary habits of an athlete, then a food diary is the best option. A food diary is simply a listing of all foods eaten over a period of time, including the type of food, preparation method, amount of food consumed, and time of consumption. This information can be input into a paper journal for analysis or directly into one of a variety of widely available computer programs. The benefit of using a computer program is it often calculates macro- and micronutrients for the provider to analyze. This method of food tracking will give the nutritional provider a more accurate accounting of the foods eaten by the athlete over a set period of time. This period of time can be anywhere from 24 hours to a full week or even ongoing. The longer the time period, the more accurate an assessment of the dietary habits of an athlete. This will provide a better picture of both macro- and micronutrient consumption as well as information about meal timing. One drawback of this type of assessment is that it heavily relies on the accuracy of the data input. An athlete who deletes meals that they feel could be considered detrimental to their progress or writes down only what will make their diet be looked on more favorably does nothing to provide accurate information to the provider. Another potential drawback could be the possibility that the athlete knows their diet is being evaluated and they could alter how they eat during the evaluation process. This would provide the nutritional practitioner with inaccurate information, leading them to draw conclusions that may not provide the benefits that the athlete is looking for. This will hurt the athlete as the analysis of the effectiveness of their diet will be based on poor information. Another concern is that the athlete feels that, since their diet is being analyzed, they are being judged for their eating habits, which could potentially lead to some concerns for disordered eating. The most important thing is for the nutritional practitioner to assure the athlete that there will be no judgment and that the food journal is only meant to obtain objective data. Additionally, the athlete should be made to feel comfortable that their data will only be used to improve their performance and that accuracy is important for this. Strong consideration should be made for the athlete to continue the journaling of their dietary intake for athletes beyond the assessment period. As an ongoing measure, this type of journaling can be used for future assessments and periodic evaluation of diet adherence. This continued journaling can act as a form of accountability for the athlete and provide possible day-to-day motivation to maintain adherence. Additionally, there has been research that demonstrates that people who record their food are more likely to be mindful of their eating due to the accountability of the journal [1]. If the athlete is going to continue a long-term food diary, I suggest they should include hydration, sleep, perceived stress levels, and performance-based information as all of this may help to guide future recommendations for both the nutritionist and the coach.

6.3.3 Food Frequency Questionnaire

A food frequency questionnaire is a tool used to try to identify trends in an athlete's dietary consumption over a given period of time, usually the weeks to months preceding the administration of the questionnaire. In a food questionnaire, the athlete would be presented with a list of foods or food categories and asked how often they were consumed daily, weekly, monthly, etc. A common follow-up to this question would be to ask the approximate serving size consumed of the food, to better assess dietary patterns. This can be done as part of the initial question, such as how often you have had a ½ cup serving of pasta in the last week, or as two separate questions. The key benefit of this type of dietary assessment is that by questioning the athlete about their consumption of specific foods, we may be able to identify consumption patterns not otherwise seen in other food intake instruments. If an athlete typically consumes Greek yogurt at a frequency of 10 servings per week but has not consumed it in the past week because the store was out of it, we may be able to note this consumption through a food frequency questionnaire when it would not show up in a food recall or even a food diary. To be more accurate, the addition of portion sizes would allow for a better assessment of how much is being consumed. A food frequency questionnaire is a good method of looking at food dietary patterns over a given time but does carry some drawbacks worth noting. One major drawback is the finite list of foods being presented in the instrument. An athlete who consumes a varied diet may find some of their typical foods to be underrepresented on the list. This would also be true of an athlete who may consume more foods identified within a specific genre (i.e., an athlete who eats a largely Mediterranean diet), which may not be captured by this instrument. A food frequency questionnaire may fail to include preparation methods, which may impact nutritional considerations. Does a food frequency questionnaire ask about deep-fried turkey? Finally, depending on how the foods are presented there is, as with all other instruments, some risk that the athlete may seek to hide what they are consuming due to the fear of being judged. This can be more common for athletes who tend to eat a diet that has less variety. A particular benefit of food frequency questionnaires is the ability to ask about alcohol, recreational drugs, and supplement use over a period of time. An athlete may have had a drink in the past 24 hours, for example, but not have had a drop of alcohol in the previous six months. This may add some context if both a food frequency questionnaire and food recall are taken together. Questions about supplement consumption are a great use of this instrument as they can help to identify their use over a longer period of time. This use may go ignored or unremembered using other tools.

In this regard, a food frequency questionnaire will help to identify factors that may impact performance that may not have otherwise been seen.

6.3.4 When to Use Dietary Assessment Instruments

A strong case should be made to use all three of the aforementioned instruments throughout your time working with athletes. Each of the aforementioned instruments provides the nutritional professional with the ability to assess the dietary habits of the athletes they work with, but each also has areas that could act as a blind spot for the athlete and leave data inaccurate. The combination of tools allows for a more complete evaluation of the athlete's true dietary habits and adherence to dietary prescriptions. This is not unlike a traditional X-ray. When a doctor orders an X-ray they order, traditionally, at least two views of the item they want to be seen. These two views, taken from differing vantage points, help to provide a more complete picture of what is going on with a patient. If you taped a quarter to the chest of a person, for example, and took a single image from the front, it would appear that the person had swallowed a quarter. Now if you then include an image taken from the side and combine the two images, it would then be clear that the quarter is above the skin. The same could be said for these dietary instruments. If an athlete eats 5000 calories in the previous 24 hours but reports an average consumption of 3000 calories daily for the past seven days, then we see that the 5000-calorie day is more likely an anomaly and may warrant further questioning as to context. If we were to look at supplementation for athletes, we can see this as well. If a presenting athlete reports that they are taking a supplement now in a food recall but not for the past six months on a food frequency questionnaire, we can get information about the impact, or lack of impact, of the supplement, particularly as some supplements may take some time to build in the system before they are effective. In this case, the addition of more than one food intake assessment allows for a more nuanced view of the overall diet when taken together.

The decision as to which of these instruments to use and when can be a highly personal one and will change based on various circumstances. The author would suggest that a food frequency questionnaire should be used for all athletes being evaluated as a means of examining long-term trends. If the athlete is making an appointment in advance, which is commonly the case, then pairing this questionnaire with a three- or seven-day food diary (the longer, the better) will provide a more complete view of dietary habits. This will give the nutritional provider an idea of what they have eaten in the past few days as well as historical averages for food intake. I tend to suggest that the food diary end at midnight before the appointment, rendering a 24-hour recall mute (or more accurately, it would be the last day of the food diary). It is not uncommon to see someone for the first time the same day as their initial contact in which case a food recall and food frequency questionnaire are very good to use in tandem. Some nutritional practitioners will ask for a food recall on all follow-up appointments, although I am more in favor of an ongoing food diary to be kept, which would make a recall unneeded as it would be included in the food diary. Although it would not be needed if they kept a diary, a food recall may be a quick assessment for follow-up appointments just to get an idea of compliance before diving into the journal. It may still be useful for an athlete if you have not had a chance to look at the journal or are keeping it digitally and looking at aggregate averages of nutrients. As stated, the combination of several of the aforementioned techniques can help to provide the nutritional practitioner a more complete understanding of the athlete's diet.

6.3.5 Indirect Calorimetry

Although not a dietary assessment, indirect calorimetry is a good tool to get an idea of the caloric needs of the client at presentation. As a nutritional provider, the ability to develop a solid nutritional strategy invariably will involve a determination of the caloric needs of the athlete. In many cases, this can be accomplished using one of several formulas available to estimate the requirements for an athlete. While these methods are clinically valuable, they are estimates used as a starting point and not a true accurate representation of the caloric output of an athlete. These formulas will be discussed in Chapter 11. Indirect calorimetry is a method to more accurately assess the actual calories used by the athlete. This process involves the measurement of both oxygen and carbon dioxide in the breath. These measurements are used to calculate the metabolic rate and the energy expenditure of the athlete. As the test involves equipment for the testing of calorimetry, this method is not one that will commonly be performed in the clinical environment [2]. If desired, an athlete can get this test performed as part of the development of an initial assessment and the information used to create a nutritional plan. As the athlete progresses, there is a need for periodic reassessment of calorimetry, although this is not going to be a frequent need. While this method is far more accurate than the equation methods, it may be overkill for many athletes to use this method and should be saved only for athletes who need this level of specificity or are not responding as expected from other methods.

6.4 Anthropometric Testing

An important part of an accurate assessment of the nutritional needs of the athlete involves the assessment of the athlete themselves. This information gives the nutritional provider information needed for utilizing macronutrient and caloric formulas. Evaluation of the presenting physical state of the athlete provides insight that can be used to guide goals, determine macronutrient needs, and even to identify areas that need to be addressed medically that may be more important than the athlete's goals. This information can also be used effectively as a means of objectively assessing the athlete's reaction to the meal planning that has been implemented. Let us take body weight as a simple example; if the nutritional provider saw an increase in performance but the body weight was climbing rapidly, there is an indication that the athlete may be putting on muscle, but the athlete may also be putting on excess body fat. This is not an inherently bad situation, but if the athlete were to put on too much body fat, there is the possibility then that the athlete's performance may suffer over a longer period of time. A deeper evaluation of the body fat percentage would be needed to help us direct the effectiveness of the dietary plan. Anthropometric testing objectively measures height, weight, circumferences, and body composition. These tests assess the structural changes accompanying training and dietary ones.

Anthropometric tests should be done at the onset of working with an athlete to help to assess the current state of their body at presentation. This information can tell the provider where the athlete is and to help with the determination of the nutritional plan. After the initial performance of anthropometric testing, they should be performed at regular intervals to provide objective data to assess the effectiveness of the nutritional plan. This data should be combined with other objective data regarding sports performance, as well as more subjective data about how the athlete is feeling while under the nutritional plan [3]. Changes to the plan should be made based on how the athlete is progressing.

6.4.1 Height

The measurement of how tall an athlete is can provide some of the basic data that can be used to determine the basal metabolic rate, body mass index, and some of the other calculations used by the nutritional practitioner. The athlete's height should be measured standing and barefoot. The measurement of height is one test that need not be repeated often as the athlete's height should not change significantly from year to year for most athletes. This is not to say that older athletes should not be remeasured as the loss of height is a good indication of skeletal conditions such as osteoporosis, and pathological bone fracture. Still, rather this assessment can be performed once per year rather than at every reexamination.

6.4.2 Weight

Body weight, in the author's opinion, may be the single most useful anthropometric measurement when working with athletes. Body weight can provide the nutritional provider with a baseline from which to base the nutritional program off. Body weight is a basic assessment of body composition that can help guide the athlete's goal setting, provide direction for the nutritional plan, and can be used to measure the outcomes of the nutritional plan. Body weight is part of the BMI assessment as well as used as part of the formulas for determining the metabolic rate and macronutrient needs for the initial nutritional strategy. This assessment should be performed at every visit and should be tracked by the athlete so that the nutritional provider may get a better insight as to the fluctuations an athlete may experience. There are many different types of scales that can be used for measuring body weight, but it is more important that the athletes be consistent in what they use to weigh themselves and, ideally, the time of day that they weigh themselves. Preferably, the athletes will weigh themselves daily first thing in the morning before they have eaten anything or had anything to drink. If body weight is measured weekly, then it should be done on the same day of the week and the same time of day to be consistent.

6.4.3 Body Measurements

Body measurements can be used for a variety of reasons as part of the nutritional assessment. They are used as part of one of the methods for measuring overall body fat. They are used as an assessment of health. They can be used as a means of monitoring progress in terms of weight loss or muscle gain. Measurements of the body are a useful tool that should be used as part of the assessment process for athletes. The measurements that I recommend monitoring include the chest at the nipple line, the waist at the navel, the hips at the widest part, the biceps, the forearm, the wrist, the neck, the thigh, and the calf. In the aforementioned cases, I would take these measurements at the initial visit and monitor them for changes monthly or bimonthly. This will give an indication of how the athlete is progressing with their nutritional strategy. The initial measurements can also be used as part of the US Navy assessment of body fat. This formula uses the athlete's age, height, weight, neck, and waist circumference to determine the approximate body fat of an athlete. This is a basic low-cost assessment of the overall body fat; while not the most accurate measure of body fat, the tape measure method is a good means of monitoring progress toward body fat goals [4]. Reductions of body fat, when measured with a tape measure, will still correlate with losses in body fat measured by other means. The waist circumference itself is a great overall assessment of health as a waist measurement of over 35 in. for females and 40 in. for males puts them into a higher risk category for cardiovascular disease [5]. The waist-to-hip measurement involves taking the waist measurement divided by the hip measurement. If the resulting number is 0.9 or higher for males and 0.83 or higher for females, then the athlete is at a higher risk for obesity-related diseases [6].

The benefits of the use of body measurements as a proxy for health are that they are inexpensive and can be done by the athlete directly or by the nutritional practitioner at every visit, if desired. The accuracy of body measurements is a drawback and the results are highly subject to the person performing the measurements, but this drawback can be reduced if you use the same person to do the measurements. Additionally, although the actual measurement may not be an ideal assessment of risk or body fat, etc., the use of multiple measurements taken over a period of time can provide the nutritional coach with accurate information if viewed from the context of change rather than absolute numbers. For example, if an athlete who desires to reduce their body fat percentage has multiple measurements performed over a three-month period showing a decline in the body fat percentage, we can assume that the nutritional plan is successful at reducing body fat even if the actual measurement is not accurate as an assessment of body fat. Let us use the waist-to-hip measurement as a further example; if the athlete presents on the first visit with a waist measurement of 50 in. and a hip measurement of 42 in., we see that their waist-to-hip measurement is 1.19, putting them in a high-risk category. After three months of nutritional intervention, this athlete now has a 40-in. waist and a 42-in. hip measurement; their waist-to-hip measurement is now 0.95, putting them at the lower end of the high-risk category. While the 0.95 number itself may not be 100% accurate, what can be inferred is that the athlete has seen a reduction in their overall risk of obesity-related diseases. I suggest that all athletes should have their comprehensive measurements taken at their initial visit so that, if nothing else, we have a baseline for when the athlete presents to the office. The nutritional provider should then determine which measurements mean the most to the athlete's goals and then repeat them at reassessments so that they can measure the progress of their nutritional interventions.

6.4.4 Body Fat Measurements

Body fat measurements are a great way for the nutritional practitioner to assist their client in achieving their performance goals. While these tests are obviously used to assess body fat and are important for athletes looking to get lean or to gain muscle without too much excess fat, they can also be used to measure the quality of weight gained, even for athletes who are less concerned with their aesthetic presentation. If, for example, an athlete working with a consultant and not gaining or losing weight, we can use a body fat analysis to see if they have experienced any changes in body composition. This information may, in some cases, be more easily seen than a change in performance. As an example, a hockey player may become leaner at the same body weight, indicating muscle gain, before they start to score more goals or win more games. In the aforementioned section on anthropometric testing, the use of body measurements for estimating body fat was discussed. In this section, further methods of body fat assessment will be explored.

6.4.5 Skinfold Caliper Measurements

The measurement of body fat using skinfold calipers provides the nutritional consultant with a method for the assessment of the body fat of the athlete. Skinfold calipers are used to measure the thickness of skinfolds as a measurement of subcutaneous body fat distribution. There are several methods that are used for measurement using different site locations and differing numbers of sites. The Durnin and Womersley method, for example, uses four sites, including the biceps, triceps, subscapular, and suprailia regions. Skinfold caliper measurement is far more accurate when compared to tape measure methods [7, 8]. Although more accurate than tape measure methods, this method is still not the most accurate method for body fat measurement. Part of the lack of accuracy is due to the inconsistencies between the individuals performing the measurements. Unlike the tape measure methods, the skinfold caliper measures cannot be done by the athletes themselves. The accuracy can be improved by having the measurements taken by the same person each time. This low-cost method, if used, should be performed at the initial assessment and at reevaluations.

6.4.6 Bioelectric Impedance Measurements

Bioelectric impedance is a simple and cost-effective method of measuring body fat for athletes. In this method, the resistance of the body to an electrical impulse is measured, after using this resistance in a standardized calculation, and this resistance is used to calculate several factors, among them body fat. Bioelectric impedance can measure the total body water, fat-free mass, and fat mass. Although a current is used, there is no pain; in fact, the person being tested cannot feel anything. This test is a low-cost method that has been included in a wide variety of devices, including scales, handheld testers, etc. The accuracy of a bioelectrical impedance device is limited by several factors, for example, obesity is sometimes poorly measured by the device. The hydration status of the athlete being tested can impact the results. Additionally, the quality of the instrument is going to affect the accuracy with a small handheld device being less accurate than a medical-grade device. A device that measures multiple points on the body, for example, will be more accurate than a simple handheld device. If using bioelectric impedance, then it is important to try to make sure the athlete is consistent with their hydration. One way to do this would be to have all assessments made under similar conditions. Although not the most accurate measurement, this low-cost method of assessing body fat is a good tool for the nutritional practitioner to use in the assessment and monitoring of athletes [9, 10].

6.4.7 Hydrostatic Weighing

Hydrostatic or underwater weighing is a method for the measurement of body fat. In this method, the athlete is submerged in a tank of water and the change in the water's height, or the displacement of water, is measured and through the use of a formula, the body fat percentage of the athlete is calculated. This method of assessing body fat composition is an accurate one but is unrealistic for use in the clinical setting. This method is often associated with research institutions, commonly associated with universities. It is unreasonable to expect a nutritional practitioner to use this method in their office, but if there is local access, then the athlete can have this test done at the start of their nutritional plan and at periodic evaluations, although less frequently than other methods [9, 10].

6.4.8 DEXA Body Fat Composition

DEXA, or dual-energy X-ray absorptiometry, is a method of assessing the body fat of an athlete. In this manner, the athlete is imaged using a specialized X-ray machine. The scans are then used to assess the body fat of the individual directly from the images. This method of assessment is very accurate compared to other tests and only moderately expensive. The in-office use of DEXA is not realistic for the nutritional practitioner, unless part of a large facility. This test is a good one to be used for accurate measurements of body fat at the start of the nutritional plan and for reevaluations [9, 10].

6.4.9 Air Displacement Body Fat Composition

Air displacement body fat analysis is a method of assessment that uses the displacement of air in an enclosed environment. In this assessment, the pressure of air is measured in an enclosed environment with the athlete. Due to the differences in the densities of differing tissues, the data obtained from the measurement can be used to estimate the fat mass and the fat-free mass. This method is not as expensive as others and is accurate. It is not common to find this type of testing environment in the clinical setting, but they are sometimes seen in large clinical settings. This is a good accurate measure of body fat testing that the nutritional practitioner can use at the outset of working with an athlete and for periodic re-evaluations [9, 10].

6.4.10 MRI and CT Body Fat Composition

Diagnostic imaging using both computed tomography and magnetic resonance imaging can be used to assess body fat. The methods use advanced imaging techniques to actually measure the body fat contained in the tissues at various sites in the body. This method is highly accurate but not inexpensive. The best application of this method is for body fat measurement in the research and to a lesser extent clinical setting. This is not an inexpensive test so like hydrostatic weighing, this is less realistic to be done in a clinical environment. This, if used by a nutritional provider, would be done at the outset of the nutritional plan and possibly periodically for reevaluation. Although accurate, the cost of these tests makes them less recommended by the author for clinical use [9, 10].

6.5 Assessments of Hydration

6.5.1 Sweat Analysis

As we have discussed, hydration plays an important role in the functional capabilities of an athlete. A dehydrated athlete will see a loss in performance as well as the potential for injury or worse. Accordingly, the hydration status of an athlete is a function of several factors ranging from water and electrolyte balance to the environment, as well as, hormonal balance. In terms of water to electrolyte balance, it is important for the athlete or anyone working with an athlete to be more aware of the quantity and qualities of the athlete's sweat. Sweat is an important function for humans to maintain homeostatic temperature balance. Heat is the byproduct of the conversion of stored energy to kinetic or movement-based energy. As we use ATP, we generate heat and the heat that is generated will raise the internal body temperature. This raise in internal temperature must be balanced as too high an internal temperature can lead to a variety of physical issues such as heat exhaustion or heat stroke. The sweating mechanism is a means of maintaining homeostatic balance by lowering the body's internal temperature through a process called convection. The sweat that makes its way to the skin is absorbed in the air as it passes across the skin, thus cooling the body. The relationship between the muscle's use of ATP to sweating can be seen clearly in terms of exercise but is also seen in the process of shivering as a means of using muscular exertion, and use of ATP, to elevate the temperature of the internal environment. As much as sweating is an essential function, with sweat, we will see the loss of vital fluids and electrolytes. This loss is not an issue if there is a balance to the losses, in other words, as long as the lost fluids and electrolytes are replaced. In order to be able to adequately plan for this, there are a variety of methods that can be employed to assess the quantity of sweat produced and the constituent makeup of the sweat produced by the athlete. A sweat analysis is a means of trying to ascertain the losses attributable to sweat so that we may be better able to develop a functional hydration plan for the athlete.

Sweat analysis seeks to determine the exact water and electrolyte needs of an athlete to better prepare to prevent the negative impacts of dehydration. There are two primary components to sweat analysis. The first is to test for the amount of sweat produced. This serves to inform the athlete or practitioner about how much water is lost by the athlete through sweat over the course of a period of time, typically a one-hour period. The second component is the sweat sodium concentration analysis, which seeks to measure the actual concentration of sodium lost during a period of exercise. There are several tests that can be used to measure both the amount and concentration of sweat lost during exercise.

6.5.2 Sweat Rate Test

A sweat rate test is a method of determining the rate at which sweat is lost over a given period of time. To determine the sweat rate, one must first determine the dry weight of an athlete prior to beginning exercise. This weight is typically taken while the athlete is naked and following urination so that only losses of fluid are noted. Nudity is important so that we may eliminate sources of fluid that may collect in the clothing. Care should be taken so that the athlete is made comfortable, as the weight is the only measurement here; the athlete can weigh themselves. A weight following exercise, for example, may be skewed by water stored in a sweaty shirt. A naked pre- and post-workout weigh-in will eliminate this source of misinformation. Following the weigh-in the athlete is then asked to perform a bout of exercise. This would be typically performed over a one-hour period. There are several schools of thought on this. If we are interested in determining a pure sweat rate, then we would pick a moderate to intense exercise but not be sport-specific (such as running on a treadmill). In the ideal scenario, we would be using the actual sport that the athlete trains in, which may give us a closer indication of how much sweat is lost during the training or performance of the specific sport for the athlete. Some variances will be encountered in an actual event due to the temperature, the nature of competition, and even differences in equipment worn (such as the equipment of a hockey player vs a runner). While the athlete is performing their bout of exercise, it is important to take note of how much fluid goes back into the body in the form of liquids consumed during athletic performance. To do this, the athlete should fill and weigh a container with the liquid they are going to consume and then after the completion of the exercise, weigh the remaining liquid noting the change in weight as the amount of liquid consumed. After exercise, the athlete will again weigh themselves both naked and having been dried with a towel to eliminate any fluids on the skin. At this point, we have the amount of weight lost (WL) during exercise (the weight before minus the weight after exercise), the weight of fluids consumed (WW), and the time of exercise. The calculation of the sweat rate (SR) would be: $SR = (WL + WW)/Time$ of exercise (see Figure 6.1).

Note: the weight lost should be converted to sweat measured in liters at a rate of 2 lbs of weight for every 1 l of sweat. Although the sweat rate can vary from athlete to athlete, we can assume that the range for sweat rate should be between 1 and 2.5 l/h. Less than 1 l/h would indicate an athlete who is not losing much fluid, assuming they are not dehydrated already. A sweat rate of over 2.5 would indicate that the athlete is losing a large amount of fluid, which must be replenished for optimal performance [11].

Figure 6.1 Sweat rate calculation.
Source: Data from Baker [11].

Sweat rate = (Weight lost + Weight of water consumed)/Time of exercise

> **Case Example**
>
> An athlete weighs 220 lbs before exercise and 215 lbs after exercise so the WL = 220 lbs − 21 lbs = 5 lbs
>
> The weight of the water bottle was 2 lbs before and 1 lb after so the WW = 2 lbs − 1 lb = 1 lb
>
> The athlete exercised for 60 minutes.
>
> $SR = (5\ lbs + 1\ lb) / 60\ minutes$
>
> $SR = 6\ lbs/h$ or $0.1\ lbs/min$
>
> $6\ lbs / 2\ lbs/l = 3\ l$
>
> The aforementioned athlete is losing approximately 3 l of fluid every hour of exercise.

As the sweat rate alone tells us nothing about the quality of the sweat the best, we can say from the aforementioned example is that the athlete is losing 3 l of fluid per hour. Assuming this number is consistent for the athlete, we can assume that they do lose a lot of sweat, which must be replenished by the athlete for optimal performance. This unfortunately does not tell us any information regarding the quality of their sweat and whether the fluid loss is purely water or more concentrated with electrolytes, specifically sodium. To accomplish this, we need to look at testing for the sweat sodium concentration.

6.5.3 Sweat Sodium Concentration

Let us look at methods for assessing the quality of the sweat loss, specifically in the loss of sodium. There are several techniques used to evaluate the concentration of sodium lost in sweat, each with its own benefits and drawbacks, mostly related to how difficult they are to perform in a clinical environment vs how accurate they are as a measurement.

The whole-body wash-down technique is the most accurate method of evaluating the amount of sodium lost in the sweat over time. To perform this test, the athlete is first washed completely in deionized water to clean and remove anything on the skin that could impair the test results. The athlete is then instructed to perform exercise over a specific interval of time. This exercise is often performed naked in an enclosed environment. Following exercise, the sweat that is released is then collected for laboratory analysis. The ability to collect a full 100% of sweat lost during exercise makes this test more accurate, but the difficulties in obtaining a sample make this test difficult, if not impossible, to perform in a clinical environment. It is for this reason that the whole-body wash down technique is most commonly seen used in research environments and is impractical for nutritional practitioners [11, 12].

A patch test is a more common test for sodium loss that can be performed clinically. This test involves the athlete performing an exercise with collection patches adhered to various points of the body. These patches can then be collected and analyzed following a bout of exercise. This patch is used as a sampling of the sweat produced by the body and can be compared to standardized samples to determine the electrolyte makeup of the sweat. This test does not collect 100% of the sweat, so the potential does exist for inaccuracy in the results; overall, it is a good assessment. The key benefit to this test is that the athlete can wear these patches and perform their sport in a more natural environment and various competition scenarios. There is no need for an athlete to exercise naked in a closed-off environment. Evaporation and contamination of the sample can present a potential for inaccurate results and must be considered. This can be minimized by performing more than one test, although this may become impractical for clinical use. The main limitation of this type of test is that it can be fairly time-consuming to analyze and therefore will limit the number of athletes who can be tested [11, 12].

6.5.4 Nonexercise Sweat Testing

A nonexercise-based sweat concentration test that has been used for cystic fibrosis patients has been increasingly used by various athletes. In this test, chemicals are applied to the athlete that would stimulate sweating with no exercise needed. This sweat can then be collected and analyzed. The benefits of this test are that there is a smaller time commitment, so more athletes can be tested. The results are reliable, but the test must also be accompanied by a sweat rate so that the concentration of the sweat can be synced with the amount of sweat lost over a period of time.

The aforementioned tests may be used as a guide for hydration planning purposes; please see Chapter 7 on hydration. The sweat test is a much more practical measure to be performed by practitioners and for most athletes needs will be enough as it helps to customize the hydration strategy. The sodium concentration tests provide important clues as to the need for electrolyte replacement during exercise but are not as practical in the clinical environment and may be best suited for advanced testing if the athlete is showing signs of dehydration despite being on a custom hydration plan.

6.6 Nutritionally Focused Lab Work

While it is beyond the scope of practice for a nutritional provider to order any lab work, there are a few laboratory tests that will help the nutritionist to make an assessment and determine their nutritional plan. The athlete will need to have these tests ordered by a provider and wither bring the results to the practitioner or have them sent directly. The following tests can help the provider to make an informed assessment.

Complete blood count with differential – this test will inform the provider of any concerns with issues concerning the immune response, the number of inflammatory cells, or any anemias that may impact performance.

Serum albumin – this measurement can help to inform the nutritional provider of the current protein status of an individual.

Vitamin and mineral blood values – these tests can inform the provider of the current state of vitamins in the athlete. While many of these vitamins are water-soluble and fluctuate rapidly, they will provide a snapshot of vitamin status and may guide the nutritional provider in crafting a plan. The concerns with B vitamins, vitamin D, iron, calcium, magnesium, potassium, and zinc are particularly important for masters athletes.

Electrolytes – these tests can inform the practitioner about the electrolyte balance at the time of presentation and may inform of any deficiencies.

High-sensitivity C-reactive protein – this biomarker for inflammation can give an indication of any issues that may inhibit recovery in athletes.

Thyroid panel – this test of T3, T4, and TSH will give an indication of any potential thyroid issues that may be of concern for the provider when creating a nutritional strategy.

Blood glucose and A1c – these tests could indicate both the potential for current concerns with blood sugar as well as an indication of long-term blood sugar control, in the case of the A1c.

Lipid profile – this test of total cholesterol, LDL, and HDL cholesterol should inform the provider of any concerns with the cardiovascular health of the individual and if there are any needs to change the nutritional plan to accommodate.

The aforementioned is not a comprehensive list of blood tests that could be performed but a sampling of the tests that may be beneficial for the nutritional provider. While the nutritional provider cannot diagnose any medical condition, an understanding of imbalances with this bloodwork may provide useful information about the current state of nutrition and anything that may potentially interfere with the nutritional strategy.

6.7 Conclusion

The assessment of the athlete is an important portion of determining the nutritional strategy. This information provides the nutritional professional information about how the athlete is currently eating, what their eating preferences look like, an indication of their current body composition, data to make estimates for the nutritional strategy, data regarding the amount of fluid they lose in their sweat to help them determine a hydration plan, and some information about the general health of the athlete. Not all of these tests can or should be done with every client, and some are outside of the scope of practice for a nutritional professional, but they all serve a purpose in the evaluation of an athlete.

References

1 Burke LE, Wang J, Sevick MA. Self-monitoring in weight loss: a systematic review of the literature. *J. Am. Diet Assoc.* 2011;111(1):92–102. doi:10.1016/j.jada.2010.10.008
2 Delsoglio M, Achamrah N, Berger MM, Pichard C. Indirect calorimetry in clinical practice. *J. Clin. Med.* 2019;8(9):1387. Published 2019 Sep 5. doi:10.3390/jcm8091387
3 Holmes CJ, Racette SB. The utility of body composition assessment in nutrition and clinical practice: an overview of current methodology. *Nutrients* 2021;13(8):2493. Published 2021 Jul 22. doi:10.3390/nu13082493
4 Shake CL, Schlichting C, Mooney LW, Callahan AB, Cohen ME. Predicting percent body fat from circumference measurements. *Mil. Med.* 1993;158(1):26–31.
5 Grundy SM, Cleeman JI, Daniels SR, et al. Diagnosis and management of the metabolic syndrome: an American Heart Association/National Heart, Lung, and Blood Institute Scientific Statement [published correction appears in Circulation. 2005 Oct 25;112(17):e297] [published correction appears in Circulation. 2005 Oct 25;112(17):e298]. *Circulation* 2005;112(17):2735–2752. doi:10.1161/CIRCULATIONAHA.105.169404
6 Murray S. Is waist-to-hip ratio a better marker of cardiovascular risk than body mass index?*CMAJ* 2006;174(3):308. doi:10.1503/cmaj.051561
7 Orphanidou C, McCargar L, Birmingham CL, Mathieson J, Goldner E. Accuracy of subcutaneous fat measurement: comparison of skinfold calipers, ultrasound, and computed tomography. *J. Am. Diet Assoc.* 1994;94(8):855–858. doi:10.1016/0002-8223(94)92363-9

8 Boughman JK, Masters MA, Morgan CA, Ruden TM, Rochelle SG. Assessing the validity of bioelectrical impedance and skinfold calipers for measuring body composition in NOLS backcountry hikers. *Wilderness Environ. Med.* 2019;30(4):369–377. doi:10.1016/j.wem.2019.06.011

9 Duren DL, Sherwood RJ, Czerwinski SA, et al. Body composition methods: comparisons and interpretation. *J. Diabetes Sci. Technol.* 2008;2(6):1139–1146. doi:10.1177/193229680800200623

10 Lemos T, Gallagher D. Current body composition measurement techniques. *Curr. Opin. Endocrinol. Diabetes Obes.* 2017;24(5):310–314. doi:10.1097/MED.0000000000000360

11 Baker LB. Sweating rate and sweat sodium concentration in athletes: a review of methodology and intra/interindividual variability. *Sports Med.* 2017;47(Suppl 1):111–128. doi:10.1007/s40279-017-0691-5

12 Baker LB, Stofan JR, Hamilton AA, Horswill CA. Comparison of regional patch collection vs. whole body washdown for measuring sweat sodium and potassium loss during exercise. *J. Appl. Physiol. (1985).* 2009;107(3):887–895. doi:10.1152/japplphysiol.00197.2009

7

Hydration

7.1 Introduction

Hydration, specifically as it relates to water, is not a major supplier of nutrients in the diet and accordingly does not immediately jump to mind when thinking about sports nutrition. This way of looking at nutrition would be a mistake, however, as hydration provides an essential component of sports performance and recovery. Hydration, or most commonly water, can often be the most overlooked element of the athlete's nutritional plan. A lack of proper hydration can have a significant negative impact on the performance of athletes, particularly older athletes. We have discussed, in Chapter 4 how macronutrients supply the energy needs for performance. Because of this, macronutrients are more likely to be viewed as the most important nutritionally when an athlete looks at consumption and utilization. Although less exciting, when compared to diet and supplementation, a lack of adequate hydration is more likely to lead to a direct negative impact on performance on the day of competition compared to, for example, a misbalanced macronutrient distribution. An athlete, for example, who consumes too little protein on the day of a competition is less likely to see as big an impact on their performance in a football game as an athlete who is dehydrated. It, therefore, stands to reason that no athlete should be overlooking the importance of proper hydration as a factor in determining their nutritional needs for maximizing performance. This chapter will examine hydration as it relates to the performance of an athlete, particularly an older athlete.

Sports Nutrition for Masters Athletes, First Edition. Peter G. Nickless.
© 2025 John Wiley & Sons, Inc. Published 2025 by John Wiley & Sons, Inc.

7.2 Water in the Body

Water comprises the single largest portion of our body weight by percent comprising around 50–60% of the total body weight. This percentage will of course change based on a variety of factors, including body composition, electrolyte balance, or age. Water is stored in two primary compartments: the first is the intracellular fluid and the second is in extracellular fluid. Intracellular fluid is the water that is found inside the cells. This water is used to provide volume and to assist with metabolic function for the cells. Extracellular fluid, on the other hand, is the amount of water found outside of the cells and comprises the water associated with the interstitial fluids such as blood plasma, lymph, and saliva. Two-thirds of all water is stored intracellularly, making it the biggest storage location for water. Water can travel into and out of the cell through semipermeable membrane that will allow the fluid to pass based on balance needs. Electrolyte and water concentrations have a lot to do with determining this balance and the flow of water into and out of the cells [1].

7.3 Functions of Water

Physiologically, water carries on many purposes in the body. The functions of water are largely based on their location in the body. If we were to look at the water found in blood plasma, for example, we see that, in this case, water is used to assist with the transportation of blood to the cells. This transportation carries importance as it is through the blood that we supply the cells with oxygen and nutrients. Additionally, we also remove metabolites and supply immune support, via white blood cells, through the blood. In this case, the role of plasma in support of athletic performance is clear. For example, nutrients are essential to athletes for, among other things, the production of energy. A decrease in blood volume can slow the delivery of these nutrients. The role of blood in supplying oxygen to tissues is also important for a variety of purposes, including aerobic energy pathways and accordingly is essential for all living creatures as well as needed for athletic performance. A decrease in blood plasma due to an altered fluid balance can result in less nutrients, oxygen, and immune cells making their way to tissues, reducing the athletic performance and recovery. Water is used and produced in various chemical reactions in the body and is therefore important to the biochemical regulation of the body processes. Water can provide structure to the cells, which in turn are important for the structural organization of the body. Water serves as an important component in the maintenance of a stable body temperature. The human body regulates temperature through several actions. When the body temperature is too low, the body will shiver to generate heat to increase temperature. When the body temperature is too high, the body will start to sweat so that the evaporation of sweat will lower the body's temperature through convection. The process of shivering involves the muscular system, and this will involve the delivery of nutrients and oxygen to the muscle tissues. It is through the body's sweat that we will see a large real-world impact of decreased water on the regulation of body temperature. A decrease in total water levels will limit the body's ability to lower the temperature and could potentially lead to overheating for an athlete. Water can play an important role in fluid-electrolyte balance in the body. Water can act as a means of helping to reduce an acidic internal environment. Proteins, to be used as buffers in the body, are transported through fluids comprises water. Functionally, water is essential to the body's ability to maintain homeostatic balance, which is needed for the survival of the athlete as well as for optimal athletic performance.

7.4 Sources of Water

As we have shown already, water is essential to survival, so the question now turns to how we get all of the water we need to carry on these processes. Water can be obtained by an individual from three primary sources. The first and most obvious source is the fluids that are consumed daily. This source includes all drinks that a person consumes throughout the day. This source of water is the largest source, accounting for approximately 80% of the water found in the body. The second source of water would be the liquid found in the food consumed as part of the diet. This amount of water is a little more difficult to assess since different foods of the same volume will contain differing levels of water content. A piece of steak cooked well done, for example, will contain much less water when compared to a similar size portion of watermelon. While not the primary source of fluid in the body, this source should be considered when making food choices. A diet rich in fruits and vegetables will contain more water, for example, than a diet low in these. The water obtained from food makes up nearly 20% of the water found in the body. The third primary source of water in the body is the metabolic water produced from various chemical reactions in the body. This water comes as a byproduct of the normal physiological reactions in the body, but the actual volume is difficult to assess [1]. This difficulty in assessing this makes it an important factor in the overall hydration status but not something that can be directly controlled or predicted by the athlete or nutritional practitioner.

7.5 Sources of Water Loss

Now that we have explored where we get water for hydration purposes, it is important to explore the ways in which we lose water. There are four primary ways in which we lose or use water. The percentages of each source of loss will be more variable and be based on factors, for example, the environmental temperature and the activity of the individual can both alter the amount of water lost daily. This demonstrates that the athlete will likely have a slightly different mix of water loss sources than the sedentary individual. The first, and most obvious source of water loss is through urination. We lose up to 2 l of fluid daily through the urinary system for most individuals. This number will vary, depending on the individual, but for most, the kidneys will remove fluids from circulation and filter it, reabsorbing the water and other chemicals that are needed to support body processes. The second most common source of daily urinary loss would be through sweat. This source of water loss will be more variable and will depend on the body's need to regulate the internal temperature, so it will be based on both environmental and activity-based factors. Logically, it can be understood that the athlete will lose more water during activities. The third source of water loss would be through defecation. This source is going to be less than urine and often less than sweat for athletes. It is important to note at this point, defecation during a bout of diarrhea, and the role of water lost in this manner, and the ability of this water loss to lead to dehydration and decreased performance. Although this is most commonly seen during periods of sickness, some athletes may have gastrointestinal issues due to anxiety and reactions to some foods. The final source of water loss for the human body would be the insensible water losses that can happen through breathing. This source of water loss will be a little more noticeable in athletes through increased respiration as well and will also increase in colder environments. The steam that escapes your mouth when breathing outside on a cold day is a good example of the water lost through breathing in cold weather [1].

7.6 Impact of Hydration Imbalance

For an athlete to achieve proper hydration, they need to be in balance between the water lost during the day and the water taken in or produced internally. This balance is essential for the athlete to be able to perform their activities without any loss in performance. The athlete will need to pay closer attention to their balance between intake and loss to avoid any imbalance. The impact of improper balance in hydration can have far-reaching effects on both the health of the individual and, as it relates to this book, sports performance. As mentioned previously, proper hydration plays a significant role in the regulation of body temperature. The inability of a dehydrated athlete to maintain their body temperature can have negative impacts on performance for the athlete. If, for example, sweat is one of the primary mechanisms we have to reduce our body temperature in a warm environment or due to exercise-related heat production, then a state of dehydration will result in a decrease in the body's ability to thermoregulate through the production of sweat. This would lead to potential cases of cramping, heat exhaustion, and heat stroke. Also, as previously discussed, the role of water balance and the regulation of cardiac output due to decreases in blood volume. This decreased blood volume can lead to increased heart rate. This increased heart rate is referred to as cardiac drift. This cardiac drift requires the heart to pump faster to deliver enough blood to fuel muscles, which can negatively impact athletic performance. Dehydration can result in decreased performance in muscular endurance and strength, as well as a decline in overall performance for the athlete. Signs and symptoms of dehydration include profuse sweating, headaches, dizziness, nausea, weakness, and even visual disturbances [2, 3]. Older athletes have an increased risk for dehydration due to the physiological changes seen with aging [4]. Fluid balance does not relate only to dehydration. Although excess fluid consumption may not be as common in athletes, it is still a case of improper fluid balance. The excess consumption of fluids, for example, can result in a potentially deadly situation called hyponatremia, which is sometimes referred to as water intoxication. The primary issue here is that an excessive increase in water consumption leads to an electrolyte imbalance, specifically when there is a decrease in sodium content. Sodium is an important electrolyte for nerve functions, cellular functions, and other various biochemical processes. Symptoms of hyponatremia can include muscle weakness, decreased coordination, disorientation, seizures, coma, and potentially even death if the condition is not treated. One example of hyponatremia seen in athletes is in those competing in endurance events where there is significant sodium loss through sweat, but replenishment is primarily water, leading to a hydration imbalance of the electrolytes and specifically low sodium content [5]. Electrolyte-infused sports drinks may help to alleviate this risk for athletes who engage in endurance activities of longer duration.

7.7 Assessing Hydration Status

Any nutritional practitioner aiming to properly hydrate an athlete to maximize performance needs to have some measure of identifying their current state of hydration status as well as some means of monitoring their hydration over time. There are several methods for assessing the hydration status of athletes; each method has benefits associated with them in relation to accuracy and ease of use. Some methods, for example, are highly accurate but are not easy to perform and therefore not reasonable for the average athlete to use on a day-to-day basis. More advanced methods of assessing hydration status, such as sweat testing and sweat sodium concentration, were discussed in more detail in Chapter 6. Other methods of assessment, such as, monitoring the athlete's body weight are relatively simple to perform but may not be as accurate when specifically looking at hydration status. To combat this, there will be some need to make a sacrifice on either accuracy or ease of use as well as this author's suggestion that multiple means be used, and their results interpreted within the context of all combined data.

The first and fastest method of assessing hydration we will discuss is the monitoring of the athlete's body weight. The monitoring of body weight is a useful tool as daily fluctuations in weight are more commonly associated with hydration and food volume status than they are true weight loss and or weight gain. In this case, however, we are specifically referring to the monitoring of body weight both before and after a workout or training session. If an athlete were to weigh 200 lbs prior to a competition and 198 lbs following the competition, then they lost 2 lbs during that athletic event; the majority of this weight would have come from water loss. If an athlete is using this method, they should plan to consume the equivalent amount of water to make up for the weight lost during athletic activity. As a rule of thumb, two to three cups of water will be needed to make up for 1 lb. of weight lost during training or competition. In the aforementioned example, four to six cups of water would be needed to make up for this loss. Depending on the sport involved and the amount of sweat lost, it may be necessary to consider an electrolyte replacement. As part of the rehydration strategy. More on this will be discussed later. Simply assessing body weight changes does carry some potential drawbacks. For example, if we just look at daily weight fluctuations, we don't take into account the impact of bladder fullness, bowel fullness, bowel habits, frequency of meals, potential water retention, and other factors. For daily weigh-ins, care must be taken to try to weigh the athletes under similar conditions. If the athlete is weighing themselves before and after a workout or competition, the impact of bladder and bowel status as well as any post-exercise eating should be taken into account as well. Another method of determining hydration status is the assessment of urine. Specifically looking at urine color, volume, and the specific gravity. Urine can be collected into a specific container and compared to a color chart which should indicate the level of hydration status. This urine can also be measured for volume as well as specific gravity measure measurements. However, these methods can be relatively accurate. They are both time-consuming and can be expensive when done daily; it is very atypical for athletes to self-analyze urine daily. One exception to this would be to simply monitor the urine for clarity as darker urine is more commonly associated with dehydration. Urine should be a clear, light amber color or lighter for proper hydration. A good argument could be made that athletes should be monitored prior to competition to determine hydration status, at least during the development phase of a hydration strategy. This could be done by a coach, athletic organization, or by the athletes themselves. In this case specifically, color and specific gravity could give an indication of how hydrated the athlete is prior to initiating activities. Potentially staving off issues with dehydration during the event and their associated health and performance risks. Combining this initial information with pre and post-exercise weighing and/or urine color examination could help to determine hydration status both at the outset of a strategy and over time.

7.8 Hydration Strategies

To ensure optimal performance for an athlete there needs to be a well-designed hydration strategy aimed at making sure there is a hydration balance. This hydration strategy needs to include both a baseline hydration plan as well as adjustments and adaptations to account for exercise induced fluid losses. On a day-to-day basis, for athletes ages 19 and above, there is a need to consume approximately 3.7 l of fluid per day for male and approximately 2.7 l of fluid per day for women. As stated previously, the sources of this fluid can come from direct drinking, the fluid in food eaten and, to a lesser degree, internally coming from metabolic activity (although this is not something that can be planned for). This is a general strategy for adult athletes, although this strategy may need to be adapted based on factors such as body composition. This does not consider the hydration needs of performance.

A good hydration strategy to maintain performance and reduce the risk of dehydration associated with exercise includes the following: a pre-exercise strategy, a strategy during the athletic event, and a post-athletic hydration strategy. Although there are many methods used, this author recommends that two to four hours before exercise begins, the athlete should consume 5–7 ml/kg of fluid. During the athletic event, the athlete should consume fluid at a rate of 0.3–2.4 ml/kg/h of sustained athletic activity. The actual

Pre-workout (2–4 hours prior)	
Fluid	5–7 ml/kg
Intra-workout	
Fluid	0.3–2.4 ml/kg
Post-workout	
Fluid	1.25–1.5 ml/kg

Figure 7.1 Hydration needs calculations. *Source:* American Dietetic Association et al. [6] and Thomas et al. [7].

amount selected will vary based on the intensity of the activity and the training environment. A post-exercise hydration strategy should include consuming approximately 1.25–1.5 ml/kg of water or fluid for every 1 lb of body weight loss during exercise, assuming the athlete has their pre-event weight [6, 7]. Although it is not generally considered a good idea to leave hydration to guesswork, if the athlete has a longstanding record of approximately how much weight they lose during an event, they may consider starting with that amount. Keep in mind that this may not suitably replenish for all cases and the athlete should re-examine this approach periodically (Figure 7.1).

There are some important considerations that must be accounted for when planning a hydration strategy for older athletes. The first consideration is the tendency toward decreased frequency of hydration at night for older adults. This is often seen as a byproduct of increased nighttime urination as one ages this is due to the changes in aldosterone and vasopressin secretion. Some older adults will decrease the amount of fluids they consume at night in an attempt to reduce the number of times they have to wake up to urinate overnight. This of course can lead to potential dehydration if fluid balance is not maintained. Aldosterone is an important hormone associated with sodium retention and as aldosterone decreases, sodium retention will also decrease. This reduction in sodium retention will lead to an increase in urinary loss. Vasopressin, sometimes referred to as antidiuretic hormone, is associated with a decrease in urination frequency. As one ages, there's a decrease in vasopressin, as well as changes in the times in which vasopressin is released, which will lead to increased urination. This can also lead to a potential source of dehydration. Another consideration when working with older adults is a decrease in thirst that is seen as people age. Additional factors that must be taken into account with older athletes are clinical issues that may impact fluid retention or loss and medication interactions that may lead to increased urination or underconsumption of fluids. Type 2 diabetes is an example of a clinical condition that is more common in older adults that may lead to increased urinary frequency and the potential for the athlete to become dehydrated. While these factors do not change the hydration needs of the athlete, they must be considered with the planning of a hydration plan for athletes.

7.9 Hydrating Sports Drinks

Sports drinks are a method employed by some athletes for the replenishment of fluid during athletic events. The beverages typically contain a combination of simple carbohydrates and electrolytes aimed at the replacement of the minerals lost during events through sweat and to provide a quick source of energy to fuel performance during the event. These drinks have value for the athlete, and the older athlete, depending on the sport and event being contested. For example, for an athlete competing in a high-intensity sport with large rest periods and a duration under 40 minutes there is rarely a need to use more than water for replenishment as carbohydrates and electrolytes can be replaced in post-workout meals. If the athlete is competing in a longer duration activity such as long-distance running, then there is often a need to refuel the athlete with carbohydrates as part of their intra workout nutritional plan and the need to replace the electrolytes lost through sweat. These athletes would benefit from a sports drink during performance. Additionally, if athletes are competing in events that have multiple sessions such as pre-season training or a tournament where there is not enough time for electrolyte replenishment between sessions, the athlete may benefit from a sports drink [8, 9]. Unfortunately, more athletes consume sports drinks than need them. Sports drinks have even become popular as a general beverage unrelated to training at all. While many sports drinks may be better for the general public than other possible drinks, they are really not doing the non-athlete or athlete in a sport that does not need a sports drink any favors. The calories alone make a sports drink that is not needed a poor choice. While it is entirely possible to include the sports drink in their macronutrient plan, it is not the most ideal use of these calories for an athlete. There are also versions of sports drinks that deviate from this mixture of carbohydrates and electrolytes either by adding extra ingredients aimed at improving performance such as caffeine or other supplements or reducing the amount of carbohydrates by providing just the electrolytes and fluid. These may have benefits in some circumstances, but the added supplements should be included only if they are part of the athlete's supplement plan, and the use of a reduced carbohydrate sports drink is best saved for situations where there is a desire to reduce calories and or sugar. One final note, despite the athletic event being performed, some environmental concerns such as high temperatures, may make the replenishment of electrolytes necessary, making sports drinks a good choice.

7.10 Conclusion

Athletic performance is reliant on a variety of factors, among them the providing and replenishment of the fluids needed for the athlete to perform at their best. Fluid balance is an important element of the athlete's nutritional plan, as the athlete must find the perfect balance between fluid intake and outtake to maintain homeostasis. A well-designed hydration strategy will allow the athlete to perform to their highest capability and recover quickly from a sporting event. A well-defined hydration plan can help prevent injury, illness, and performance loss due to dehydration. This has particular importance for master's athletes as they are more prone to becoming dehydrated when compared to younger athletes.

References

1 Brinkman JE, Dorius B, Sharma S. Physiology, body fluids. [Updated 2023 Jan 27]. In: StatPearls [Internet]. Treasure Island (FL): StatPearls Publishing, 2024. Available from: https://www.ncbi.nlm.nih.gov/books/NBK482447/
2 Winger JM, Dugas JP, Dugas LR. Beliefs about hydration and physiology drive drinking behaviours in runners. *Br. J. Sports Med.* 2011;45(8):646–649. doi:10.1136/bjsm.2010.075275
3 Maughan RJ, Shirreffs SM. Dehydration and rehydration in competitive sport. *Scand. J Med. Sci. Sports* 2010;20 Suppl 3:40–47. doi:10.1111/j.1600-0838.2010.01207.x
4 Soto-Quijano DA. The competitive senior athlete. *Phys. Med. Rehabil. Clin. N. Am.* 2017;28(4):767–776. doi:10.1016/j.pmr.2017.06.009
5 Von Duvillard SP, Braun WA, Markofski M, Beneke R, Leithäuser R. Fluids and hydration in prolonged endurance performance. *Nutrition* 2004;20(7–8):651–656. doi:10.1016/j.nut.2004.04.011
6 American Dietetic Association; Dietitians of Canada; American College of Sports Medicine, Rodriguez NR, Di Marco NM, Langley S. American College of Sports Medicine Position Stand Nutrition and athletic performance. *Med. Sci. Sports Exerc.* 2009;41(3):709–731. doi:10.1249/MSS.0b013e31890eb86

7 Thomas DT, Erdman KA, Burke LM. American College of Sports Medicine Joint Position Statement. Nutrition and Athletic Performance [published correction appears in Med Sci Sports Exerc. 2017 Jan;49(1):222]. *Med. Sci. Sports Exerc.* 2016;48(3):543–568. doi:10.1249/MSS.0000000000000852

8 Vitale K, Getzin A. Nutrition and supplement update for the endurance athlete: review and recommendations. *Nutrients* 2019;11(6):1289. Published 2019 Jun 7. doi:10.3390/nu11061289

9 Orrù S, Imperlini E, Nigro E, et al. Role of functional beverages on sport performance and recovery. *Nutrients* 2018;10(10):1470. Published 2018 Oct 10. doi:10.3390/nu10101470

8

Peri-workout Nutrition

8.1 Introduction

To this point, this book has focused primarily on how the athlete needs to fuel themselves over the course of their day, little attention, however, has been spent on nutrient timing for optimal performance. This is where the concept of peri-workout nutrition comes in. Peri-workout nutrition refers to the nutrition that the athlete will utilize before, during, and after the workout to optimize their ability to perform their athletic events and to recover from them. While the total nutritional intake for the day is more important for the athlete to get correct, the topic of peri-workout nutrition can provide the finishing touches by applying the nutrients directly around the time period when the athlete needs them the most. This focus on sports nutrition allows us to target energy to the time period where it will impact performance and recovery the most. This subject has quite a few different approaches, but we will discuss some effective ways of approaching peri-workout nutrition. Peri-workout nutrition covers the nutritional needs of the athlete before (pre-workout) during (intra-workout) and after (post) their workout or competition. These three phases are all important but for different reasons. It is important to also consider the sport being contested or trained for. A skill-based activity, for example, often does not tax the energy systems beyond what could be replenished during a normal day of eating and often will not require a peri-workout nutritional plan. Target shooting, for example, is a sport that does not have the energy demands of an activity that would require peri-workout nutrition. Although a difficult activity, and one worthy of acclaim, it does not have the same demand on the body as a more intense activity in that optimal performance requires energy needs be replenished during the event or immediately after. It is also important to point out that, for the most part, the macronutrients consumed

Sports Nutrition for Masters Athletes, First Edition. Peter G. Nickless.
© 2025 John Wiley & Sons, Inc. Published 2025 by John Wiley & Sons, Inc.

during the peri-workout period are not in addition to the pre-determined macronutrient needs but come from them, suggesting that peri-workout nutrition is more about nutrient timing. An athlete who is suggested to consume 500 g of carbohydrate daily, and 120 g of this is suggested peri-workout, would only have 380 g for the rest of the day. Peri-workout nutrition is about how we time the nutrients to assist the athlete to achieve their optimal performance.

8.2 Pre-workout Nutrition

Pre-workout nutrition refers to the nutritional needs of the athlete before they engage in either training or competitive activity. The primary goal of pre-workout nutrition would be to provide the fuel the athlete needs to perform either training or competition and should focus on providing the nutrients needed for the athlete to be able to succeed in their event. The focus is to provide energy, improve endurance, improve performance, and reduce muscle breakdown which will enhance performance for athletes. The first thing the author suggests for establishing a pre-workout nutritional plan would be to consume about 20–30 g of protein [1]. The purpose of this would be for blood sugar control as well as the potential anabolic response which could help to support the athlete. Protein plays an important role in reducing the impact on blood sugar for the athlete; if the athlete were to consume carbohydrates alone, they could see a spike in blood sugar, which could result in a crash during the event. Protein helps to blunt this response, keeping blood sugar stable. The next thing that the athlete will need is carbohydrates. The purpose of these carbohydrates is to satisfy some of the energy needs the athlete will have as they start performing their upcoming activity. These carbohydrates should ideally be of a lower glycemic type, as this will provide a more sustained energy boost over the ensuing time. The recommendation would be for the athlete to consume 1–2 g of carbohydrates per kilogram of body weight [1]. Therefore, a 100 kg athlete should consume between 100 and 200 g of carbohydrate before their athletic event. The actual amount will depend on the event being trained for or contested and the energy requirements of the event. If the athlete were competing in a baseball game, they would be suited to an amount closer to 100 g due to the lower energy requirements of the sport. An endurance runner, on the other hand, would be better suited for 200 g, using the aforementioned example, as their sport will have a more constant need for energy. One important consideration for pre-workout nutrition would be the need to time the consumption of these nutrients to allow the athlete to digest and perform. Some athletes find that food consumed within an hour of athletic activity is too much for their digestive system and can have a negative impact on their performance. Another consideration would be how the athlete performs with pre-workout carbohydrates. The event being contested may support 2 g/kg of body weight, but if the athlete finds they are sluggish and do not perform well at 200 g, but they do perform better with 100 g, then that would be better for the athlete. It is always important to note that although these guidelines will work for most athletes, the nutritional practitioner or coach needs to always consider feedback and input from the athlete regarding how they feel or perform with these interventions. This is an area where experience working with, and listening to athletes will make a difference. Having the athletes keep a journal where they report this pre-workout consumption and how they feel afterward will help inform the practitioner on how to adjust the plan.

8.2.1 Reactive Hypoglycemia

One concern when preparing athletes for competition would be the ideal timing for pre-event carbohydrates, particularly high glycemic carbohydrates. While on one hand, we know that carbohydrates fuel performance, particularly in endurance events, they can also lead to a problem known as reactive hypoglycemia. Reactive hypoglycemia can have the opposite of the desired effect of consuming pre-workout carbohydrates and reduce performance as the body tries to overcome the symptoms associated with the rapid changes in blood sugar. With reactive hypoglycemia, the ingestion of a large amount of carbohydrates, often within two hours of the event, can lead to a dramatic rise in blood sugar. The reaction to this elevation in the athlete's blood sugar is to release insulin in an attempt to lower blood sugar by removing the excess sugar from the blood (typically for storage in the liver and muscles as glycogen). The issue with this, however, is that when this happens before exercise, there is often a lowering of blood sugar below the levels needed to perform the sport in question, leading to limitations in performance for the athlete. Symptoms of reactive hypoglycemia can include anxiety, confusion, sweating, increased heart rate, irritability, shaking, lightheadedness, and fainting [2, 3]. To prevent reactive hypoglycemia from happening, it is best for the athlete to focus the consumption of carbohydrates to more than two hours before an event and even to try to limit pre-event carbohydrates to those that are lower on the glycemic index. Additionally, the consumption of proteins and fats in addition to carbohydrates will reduce the impact of the insulin response for the athlete thus reducing the risks from reactive hypoglycemia before an athletic event.

There is also a risk of reactive hypoglycemia during an event if the glycogen levels fall too low. To avoid this reactive hypoglycemia, the athlete must prepare for the event by using adequate peri-workout nutrition. As there is an increased risk of reactive hypoglycemia for those with diabetes and prediabetes, particularly for those taking medications, there is an increased need to be concerned with this for those working with older athletes who are at a greater risk of insulin balance conditions [3].

8.2.2 Carbohydrate Loading

The prevailing limitation for athletes looking to perform their athletic activities to the fullest is the ability for them to be able to replenish the ATP needed to perform their athletic events during competition or training. This would indicate that for most sports, the substrate used primarily by the energy systems involved in the athletic event would be the limiting factor. For many events, this will boil down to intensity and duration. A high-intensity activity, for example, is more likely to use carbohydrates as a primary fuel source, indicating the ability to perform optimally in this activity will be influenced by the amount of carbohydrates available to the athlete. In many athletic cases, the largest source of stored energy for use by the athletes will come from the glycogen stored in the liver and, most importantly, the muscle. After this glycogen is used then, attention will turn to the replacement of energy from the nutrition consumed by the athlete during their event. This leads many in the field to, understandably, want to focus on maximizing the glycogen stored in the muscle prior to the event as a means of maximizing available energy sources to the athlete. This is the basis behind the concept of carbohydrate loading, the ingestion of larger-than-normal amounts of carbohydrates before an event with the goal of maximizing energy stores to be used in the event. This carbohydrate loading can be done in different ways, ranging from a basic high-carbohydrate meal prior to the event to a highly scientific approach to maximize carbohydrate storage potential. Carbohydrate loading duration can take a single meal the night before all the way up to three days prior to the event. The athlete is consuming a larger than normal amount of carbohydrate during this time containing approximately 8–10 g/kg of bodyweight [4, 5]. This would mean that a 100 kg athlete would consume up to 1200 g of carbohydrates the day before a competition. One goal of focusing the carbohydrates to the period before the event is to attain something called supercompensation. Supercompensation is when the glycogen stores are temporarily swelled to accommodate more glycogen than they would normally contain. This cannot be maintained, but proponents feel that this will give the athlete an advantage in competition as they will have more energy available for use. The strategies of carbohydrate loading are not as effective for shorter duration sports as the athlete very commonly has enough stored glycogen from normal daily eating to accommodate the energy needs of the sport. A sprinter, a weightlifter, and a football player, for example, will not see a major performance improvement from carb loading. There is some evidence that suggests longer-duration athletes would see a benefit with carb loading supported by a good intra-workout nutritional plan. These athletes would be those competing in sports like long-distance running, cycling, ironman, and half-ironman length triathlons. In terms of carbohydrate loading and older athletes, there is little evidence indicating that this strategy will not work for appropriate athletic events, in the absence of any condition or disorder that would impact carbohydrate metabolism or insulin control. Food choice is a consideration for carbohydrate loading strategies, although this is more of a long-term health issue than a sports performance one as research indicates the choice of carbohydrate has little to do with the impact on performance for carbohydrate loading. As insulin control and long-term health are important to athletes of all ages, it is suggested that carbohydrate-loading strategies include more foods that are lower on the glycemic index and include more complex carbohydrates [6, 7]. One thousand grams of table sugar, for example, will have a large impact on insulin secretion and potential negative impacts on overall health when compared to fruits and vegetables with a lower glycemic index. For some sports that will rely heavily on glycogen as a fuel source, carbohydrate loading can be an effective strategy for maximizing performance.

8.3 Intra-workout Nutrition

The nutrition we use to fuel the workout during training or in competition is referred to as intra-workout nutrition. The focus of intra-workout nutrition is predominantly carbohydrate replenishment to maintain performance as the athlete has started to use up the stored glycogen and carbohydrates circulating in the blood. In this case, we need to consider not only the size of the athlete and the sport being engaged in but also the length of the training or competitive event being contested. Athletes who are contesting sports that last less than 30 minutes do not need to consider any carbohydrate replenishment during the workout [1]. They should have enough stored glycogen to satisfy the needs of the event. This may be in stark contrast to some commonplace scenes of athletes in your local gym drinking a sports carbohydrate drink during a routine fitness workout. This is likely not needed and even, in the event that the workout goes longer than 30 minutes, is still likely overkill based on the nutritional needs of their particular workout. Additionally, if the athlete is looking to control their body weight, then this source of, likely, unnecessary calories could be detrimental to their goal. If the sport lasts over thirty minutes, then the athlete should consume between 30 and 60 g of carbohydrates per hour in order to ensure the athlete's ability to maintain performance levels as they train or compete. This would mean that a runner doing a one-hour run would be looking to take in around 30–60 g of carbohydrates; the actual amount would be based on intensity or duration, as a higher intensity may lean toward the 60 g of carbohydrate recommendation. After the first hour of training or competition, the athlete should consume an additional 30–60 g of carbohydrate per hour [1]. The form of this carbohydrate should be more of a simple carbohydrate that is quick and easy to digest, such as a glucose or sucrose-based drink. Carbohydrate gels and gummies are also used for this use and often contain a similar type of sugar that is fast to digest. Although fructose can be used to fuel this performance some athletes will find that too much. Fructose can lead to gastrointestinal discomfort for some athletes which can have a negative impact on performance. If choosing to get some of these carbohydrates in drinkable forms (such as a powder or electrolyte replacement drinks), it is recommended that the mixture be more dilute in warmer environments where dehydration is more of a concern. In more mild temperatures, there is no need for dilution of carbohydrate drinks. It is only after three or more hours (less if training or competing in a hot environment) that electrolyte replenishment needs to be considered. The likelihood that the athlete will need to replace their electrolytes quickly during a two-hour event in moderate temperatures is much lower than during a three- to four-hour sporting event and can often be accomplished through their normal dietary consumption [1]. Again, this should be reevaluated in environments where the athlete is sweating more due to the heat and electrolyte replacement should be considered earlier in the event. As with pre-workout nutrition, the athlete's performance should be monitored, and the intra-workout reevaluated.

8.4 Post-workout Nutrition

After the event or training is completed, it is important that the athlete focus on post-workout nutrition to start the process of refueling, recovering, and repairing tissues immediately. The goal of this is to replenish nutrients used during the athletic performance and to assist in recovery and refuel for future performance. Some studies have shown that the hour post-workout

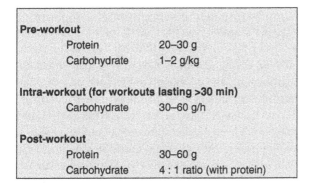

Figure 8.1 Peri-workout nutrition. *Source:* Kerksick et al. [1], Pritchett and Pritchett [8], and Schoenfeld et al. [10].

anabolic window or "golden hour" is an important repair and rebuilding time and the nutrition taken in during this time is essential for recovery. This post-exercise "golden hour" does not have universal acceptance with studies questioning the need for the refeed, and some even suggesting the pre-workout consumption of protein and the workout itself will provide enough stimulation for muscle protein synthesis [8, 9]. This book is less focused on an idealized anabolic window than the need to refuel and recover, preparing the athlete for the next workout; therefore, the author still recommends a post-workout meal. Protein, essential for muscle repair and growth, should be consumed at 20–30 g in the first 30 minutes ideally. Carbohydrates should be consumed in that same time period in a 4:1 ratio or 60–120 g [8, 10]. There is a recovery benefit of having a higher glycemic carbohydrate during this time. The athlete should resume their normal eating plan after this post-workout meal. Nutritional practitioners need to assess and alter the post-workout nutritional plan based on subsequent performance and athlete perception of their progress toward goals (Figure 8.1).

8.5 Conclusion

The need for the athlete to fuel optimal performance necessitates an increased focus on the timing of their nutrition surrounding the athletic event. Although a solid nutritional plan should be suitable for most athletes to perform their activities a focused peri-workout nutritional plan is going to ensure the delivery of nutrients at the time the athlete most needs it. Additionally, when we look at longer-duration sports, such as long-distance running, the role of peri-workout nutrition goes beyond optimal performance to being outright essential to the athlete's ability to perform the requirements of their sport. An ultra-runner, for example, may find that their performance, and ability to even finish an event, absolutely depends on their consumption of nutrition during the event. The development of a solid peri-workout nutritional plan will provide the athlete with the nutrients needed to support their athletic endeavors and to perform at their best. It should be noted that the focus of this chapter has been the determination of nutrient requirements for peri-workout nutrition. Peri-workout nutrition can include a combination of both whole food and supplements; in many cases, supplements may be preferable for athletes as it may be easier for an athlete to consume a drink to get their carbohydrates rather than to eat during an event. The use of pre-workout stimulant-based supplements was not discussed in this chapter as they are less about providing the athlete with the nutrients needed to perform their events, but rather, they are used for their performance-enhancing benefits. These pre-workout supplements will be discussed in more detail in Chapter 10.

References

1 Kerksick CM, Arent S, Schoenfeld BJ, et al. International Society of Sports Nutrition Position Stand: nutrient timing. *J. Int. Soc. Sports Nutr.* 2017;14:33. Published 2017 Aug 29. doi:10.1186/s12970-017-0189-4
2 Altuntaş Y. Postprandial reactive hypoglycemia. *Sisli Etfal Hastan Tip Bul.* 2019;53(3):215–220. Published 2019 Aug 28. doi:10.14744/SEMB.2019.59455
3 Brun JF, Dumortier M, Fedou C, Mercier J. Exercise hypoglycemia in nondiabetic subjects. *Diabetes Metab.* 2001;27(2 Pt 1):92–106.
4 Noakes TD. What is the evidence that dietary macronutrient composition influences exercise performance? A narrative review. *Nutrients* 2022;14(4):862. Published 2022 Feb 18. doi:10.3390/nu14040862
5 Sedlock, DA. The latest on carbohydrate loading: a practical approach. *Curr. Sports Med. Rep.* 2008;7(4):209–213. doi:10.1249/JSR.0b013e31817ef9cb
6 Strasser B, Pesta D, Rittweger J, Burtscher J, Burtscher M. Nutrition for older athletes: focus on sex-differences. *Nutrients* 2021;13(5):1409. Published 2021 Apr 22. doi:10.3390/nu13051409
7 Rothschild JA, Kilding AE, Plews DJ. What should I eat before exercise? Pre-exercise nutrition and the response to endurance exercise: current prospective and future directions. *Nutrients* 2020;12(11):3473. Published 2020 Nov 12. doi:10.3390/nu12113473

8 Pritchett K, Pritchett R. Chocolate milk: a post-exercise recovery beverage for endurance sports. *Med. Sport Sci.* 2012;59:127–134. doi:10.1159/000341954

9 Aragon AA, Schoenfeld BJ. Nutrient timing revisited: is there a post-exercise anabolic window? *J. Int. Soc. Sports Nutr.* 2013;10(1):5. Published 2013 Jan 29. doi:10.1186/1550-2783-10-5

10 Schoenfeld BJ, Aragon A, Wilborn C, et al. Pre-versus post-exercise protein intake has similar effects on muscular adaptations [published correction appears in PeerJ. 2017 Aug 1;5]. *PeerJ* 2017;5:e2825. Published 2017 Jan 3. doi:10.7717/peerj.2825

9

Inflammation

9.1 Introduction

Inflammation, or more accurately, the inflammatory process, refers to a series of complex biochemical processes that are essential in helping the body to battle infection, heal from exercise, or protect and repair itself following an injury. The issue associated with inflammation in relation to athletic performance is not the impact that the typical inflammatory process has but rather the control of this process from overreaction to a stimulus. The inflammatory process consists of a series of biochemical pathways that modulate the response to infection or injury. The pathways can have direct, immediate, and acute impacts as well as chronic, more long-term impacts that can have a role in the overall health and the performance of the athlete. A big misconception is that inflammation is something that should be eliminated; the inflammatory process is a protection mechanism that is necessary for maintaining homeostasis. It is not only impossible but detrimental to eliminate inflammation from the life of an athlete. The bigger concern is that, in some cases, the inflammatory process can become overstimulated and lead to a negative impact for the athlete in terms of both health and athletic recovery and performance. There are nutritional and lifestyle factors that can be modified to provide the athlete with the best chance of limiting the overall inflammatory response, allowing the athlete the ability to recover and perform to their best. This chapter will examine the physiology of the inflammatory response as well as the role of nutrition and lifestyle modification in mediating inflammation.

9.2 The Physiology of Inflammation

In order to manage and potentially control the inflammatory response in athletes, it is essential that the nutritional provider have an understanding of the physiology involved with the inflammatory response. The first part of the inflammatory response is the introduction of a stimulus that would start the process. The goal of the inflammatory process is to recognize this stimulus, eliminate the stimulus, and repair any damage caused by the stimulus. This stimulus can be from a variety of sources. An intense bout of exercise is an example of a stimulus that can initiate the inflammatory response, as is a cut, a strain, a poor diet, lack of sleep, etc. The response to this stimulus is the release of inflammatory chemicals to stimulate the dilation of blood vessels, including histamine, prostaglandins, and cytokines. Histamine, released from the mast cells acts on the blood vessels by dilating them. Prostaglandins support the vasodilation of the blood vessels as well as play a role in pain sensation. The cytokine chemicals assist in regulating the release of inflammatory cells to the site of the stimulus. This dilation leads to an increase in blood flow to the site of the stimulus to bring with it inflammatory cells (particularly neutrophils and macrophages), oxygen, and nutrients. This increase in blood flow will lead to the area becoming red and warm to the touch. At the site of the stimulus the vessels become increasingly permeable to allow the inflammatory cells and fluid to enter the area. This, particularly the release of the inflammatory white blood cells, is an attempt to neutralize the threat by killing any foreign pathogens or cleaning up the area. This release of fluid and inflammatory cells to the area is seen by the symptom of swelling. As a result, to the cellular response, more chemicals, namely tumor necrosis factor-alpha, interleukins, and leukotrienes, are released that enhance the inflammatory response, recruiting even more cells to the area. Once there is control of the stimulus, the inflammatory response begins to slow down. Anti-inflammatory chemicals, e.g., glucocorticoids and anti-inflammatory cytokines, are released to help with the slowdown of the inflammatory process. At this time, the body begins to clean up the area, using macrophages, as well as repair the damage caused by the inflammation.

9.2.1 Acute and Chronic Inflammation

The inflammatory process can be both acute, dealing with short-term quick reactions to stimuli, or chronic, which has a more long-term response to the stimuli. A sprained ankle is an example of an acute injury, and the acute response is the short-term actions taken to respond to this stimulus, stop the progression, and repair the damage caused by the stimulus. The acute response acts quickly to respond to the stimulus, but the reaction does not last long often days to a few weeks in duration. Redness, swelling, heat, and pain tend to accompany the acute response as seen earlier. The goal of the acute inflammatory response is to eliminate and heal the stimulus as quickly as possible. A chronic inflammatory response on the other hand is a more long-term approach. This response does not have the same speed of response nor is the response as great as compared to acute inflammation. Chronic inflammation responds more to ongoing stimuli such as chronic infections, poor diet, or chronic exposure to environmental irritants, such as smoking. While acute inflammation is often resolved in a matter of weeks, chronic inflammation can last much longer often for months or even years. Long-term chronic inflammation can impact the blood vessels and other organs, increasing the chances of chronic diseases. If left untreated or unresolved, the acute inflammatory response has the potential to become a more long-term chronic response. While most athletes deal with acute inflammation in the form of sports injuries, athletes, particularly master's athletes, who have accumulated a lifetime of injuries and or stimuli, are also affected by chronic inflammatory processes. Both of these processes are essential to maintaining homeostasis but must be controlled and kept from expanding for optimal performance and recovery.

9.3 Inflammation in Athletes

Now that we have discussed a little about the inflammatory process as well as the differences between acute and chronic inflammation, we will now examine some of the common causes and sources of inflammation that athletes will encounter. Athletes like all people are at risk for acute injuries resulting in inflammation. These sources are well known and include sprain, strains, muscle tears, and cuts. While these are important considerations, more exploration is needed into the nontraumatic sources of inflammation. Some common sources of inflammation for athletes include the inflammation caused by the exercises themselves, the diet of the athlete, and environmental risk factors that lead to inflammation.

9.3.1 Exercise

The act of performing an exercise, and the overall load of exercise in general, leads to a low-level inflammation as a result of the microdamage caused by the athletic activity. As part of the exercise process, the body experiences a small amount of microtrauma that mobilizes the inflammatory response. This response triggers the acute inflammatory process outlined earlier. Part of the typical recovery process after exercise involves the increase and resolution of the inflammatory process. Typically, with enough rest, the athlete is able to see the inflammatory response through to its resolution. Inflammation of this nature is part of the recovery process and how athletes progress from training. The problem occurs when the acute inflammation from exercise is not allowed to fully resolve before engaging in more exercise. This prolonged exposure to the microtrauma can lead to a more chronic inflammatory state. As the athlete ages, the inflammatory response is slowed overall, often due to the cumulative inflammatory response in the whole body. This tends to lead to a more chronic low-grade inflammation and a longer time for the athlete to recover between bouts of exercise. A well-designed exercise routine with proper rest, nutrition, and hydration can help to reduce the impact of exercised-induced inflammation.

9.3.2 Nutrition and Inflammation

Diet plays a role in the inflammatory response; diet can exacerbate the inflammatory response and trigger inflammation. A food can act as a stimulus, leading to the initiation of the inflammatory response. If this dietary exposure was singular, the body would often be able to recover from the inflammation. Unfortunately, often with dietary issues, the athlete has eaten an inflammatory food that has initiated a response, but rather than ending the response, they continue to eat the same foods, propagating the response and turning it from an acute to a chronic inflammation. Often this is because the initial stages of the response have no overt symptoms. Foods that promote inflammation, or pro-inflammatory foods, are those that have been shown to act as stimuli and activate the inflammatory processes. These foods trigger the response and increase production of cytokines, prostaglandins, and leukotrienes. Long-term consumption of these foods leads to a chronic low-grade inflammation and can impact recovery from exercise as well as contribute to long-term chronic diseases, such as cardiovascular disease. Pro-inflammatory foods that can increase the inflammatory response include processed foods, such as processed cereals or meats; refined foods, such as white bread and baked goods high in sugar; sugar-sweetened beverages, trans fats, saturated fats, omega-6 fatty acids; and some food additives [1]. Additionally, in some athletes, there is an individual response to foods that can make a food that is perfectly acceptable for some pro-inflammatory for other people. Care should be taken when designing diets for athletes to avoid these foods.

9.3.3 Environment and Inflammation

The environment that the athlete lives in and the air the athlete breaths have the capability of stimulating the inflammatory response in a manner similar to how foods can enhance it. Factors that can lead to an inflammatory response include air pollution, from factories or car exhaust, exposure to toxins and chemicals, such as cleaning chemicals, PCBs, pesticides, and heavy metals, changes in temperatures, extremes in heat and cold, and lifestyle factors such as smoking drinking, drugs, etc. Stress is an example of a potential source of inflammation that is not the external environment but the internal environment. Stress acts as a trigger for the inflammatory response, but left unchecked, this stress can turn an acute issue into a more chronic problem. This is a particular concern for athletes, as they are often dealing with the stresses of competition, training, relationships, finances, lack of sleep, etc. Stress has impacts beyond the immune response. Stress can impact the endocrine system through the release of excess cortisol, the activation of the sympathetic fight or flight response, and disruption in the gut microbiome. All of which can enhance the inflammatory response. These factors are often difficult to control, for example, an athlete living in a major city may not be able to avoid breathing the exhaust of vehicles in traffic. Care must be taken to limit or eliminate the exposure to these potential irritants whenever possible. While this is strictly not a nutrition subject, the nutritionist can identify sources of environmental exposure through a thorough history of the athlete and their lifestyle.

9.4 Managing Inflammation for Performance

We have discussed the factors that can lead to an increase in the inflammatory process for an athlete. We discussed the impact of the exercise regime and how it can impact inflammation. We discussed lifestyle factors such as sleep, alcohol, drugs, etc. and how they can lead to a chronic low-grade inflammation. Most importantly, we discussed the role that diet can play in inflammation, particularly how a poor diet can lead to an exacerbation of a low-grade inflammatory state. In this section, we will discuss how dietary changes, supplementation, and targeted recovery techniques can be used by the athlete to limit the impact of the inflammatory process and its impact on sports performance.

9.4.1 Dietary Strategies to Reduce Inflammation

9.4.1.1 Reduce Sources of Inflammation from the Diet

As we examine the dietary strategies to support the regulation and potential limitation of the inflammatory process, we can see two primary strategies emerging. The first strategy is the limitation of the pro-inflammatory foods that are consumed. As discussed, these foods act as a stimulus starting the inflammatory process and if consumed repeatedly, or in amounts that are above what the body can deal with, then the short-term stimulus becomes more of a long-term chronic one. The first solution to this is to eliminate these sources of inflammation from the diet. This means that the nutritional strategies employed need to reduce the amount of processed foods in the diet, reduce the overall consumption of sugar and refined carbohydrates, and eliminate the excess omega-6 fatty acids in the diet [2]. Additionally, feedlot-fed animals can be a source of pro-inflammatory food in the diet [3, 4]. The elimination of these pro-inflammatory stressors can help reduce a significant amount of inflammation but may fall short of eliminating all potential stressors. This should always be the first step.

If the athlete has any foods that may be a problem for them due to allergies, etc., a more detailed approach would also look to eliminate these sources as well. The two methods to recognize these foods are the low-tech eliminate and challenge method and laboratory analysis. In the eliminate and challenge method a food is eliminated for a period of time, often 21 days, and then reintroduced to see any subjective or objective changes noted by the athlete such as pain, bloating, and GI stress. This testing has the advantage of being low-cost and easy to implement for a nutritional professional, but there is a major time commitment involved in finding the issue. Laboratory analysis, on the other hand, can be quickly and easily performed and trigger foods identified for potential exclusion from the diet. One negative aspect of this approach is that for most nutritional professionals, ordering lab work will be beyond their legal scope of practice and testing needs to be done by an appropriate professional. These tests can also be expensive, which can be an additional barrier. With this in mind, the removal of known pro-inflammatory foods should be the first consideration with advanced evaluations for specific food triggers to be examined if the desired effects are not achieved.

9.4.1.2 Increase the Consumption of Anti-inflammatory Foods

After the elimination of foods that are known to trigger an inflammatory reaction, we must consider the addition of foods that have been demonstrated to have properties that reduce inflammation. An anti-inflammatory food is one that has properties that act to antagonize the aforementioned inflammatory processes. Let us look, for example, at foods rich in omega-3 fatty acids; these foods can help to inhibit the production of the pro-inflammatory prostaglandins and leukotrienes mentioned earlier. Additionally, EPA and DHA in omega-3 fatty acids contain specialized pro-resolving mediators that can help to reduce inflammation as well as repair tissue. In this case, the impact of omega-3-rich foods can have a potentially beneficial effect of the diet [5–7] Anti-inflammatory foods fall into several categories omega-3 fatty acids, antioxidant-rich foods, anti-inflammatory herbs, and spices examples of which can be found in the following text.

Omega-3 fatty acids [5–7]
- **Fatty fish** – salmon, mackerel, sardines, trout, and tuna
- **Shellfish** – assuming the athlete has no allergies
- **Plant-based sources** – walnuts, chia seeds, flax seeds, canola oil, hemp seeds, and soybeans

Antioxidant-rich foods [5–7]
- **Fruits** – berries, cherries, citrus fruits, etc.
- **Vegetables** – green leafy vegetables, broccoli, beets, tomatoes, etc.
- **Nuts and seeds** – almonds, walnuts, Brazil nuts, pecans, etc.
- **Whole grains** – oats, barley, quinoa, brown rice, etc.
- **Legumes** – beans, lentils, peas, etc.

Anti-inflammatory herbs and spices [5–7]
- Turmeric
- Ginger
- Cinnamon
- Garlic
- Cloves
- Rosemary
- Oregano
- Basil
- Thyme
- Sage
- Cilantro
- Peppermint
- Fennel
- Dill
- Onion

While an exhaustive list of all of the anti-inflammatory foods and their preparation methods is beyond the scope of a sports nutritional professional and this book, the incorporation of the aforementioned foods can help the athlete to reduce some of the inflammatory reactions. Whenever possible the athlete should strive to consume the aforementioned foods in their whole food form, particularly using fresh herbs and spices when possible.

9.4.2 Supplementation to Reduce Inflammation

While ideally much of the heavy work in reducing inflammation will come from eliminating the pro-inflammatory foods and increasing the anti-inflammatory foods, supplementation can be a good supportive aid for gaps in supporting the goal of reducing inflammation. The supplements that can help support the reduction of inflammation will be discussed in Chapter 10 but include:

Anti-inflammatory supplements [8–10]
- **Omega 3 fatty acids** – from fish oils or plant sources
- **Curcumin** – from turmeric
- Boswellia serrata
- Probiotic supplements
- Quercetin
- Tart cherry
- Vitamin D
- Magnesium

This is not an exhaustive list of all of the supplements with anti-inflammatory properties, but there are some supplements commonly used by athletes to support dietary changes aimed at reducing inflammation.

9.4.3 Recovery Techniques to Reduce Inflammation

In addition to the aforementioned nutritional strategy, several recovery techniques could be employed to support the athlete as they look to control the inflammatory process. While these techniques are not nutrition, they do support the master's athlete in achieving their goals and work alongside a well-designed nutritional plan to help control inflammation. In addition to nutrition, proper hydration will play an important role as hydration is needed to support the cellular processes that participate in the inflammatory reactions as well as prevent any inflammation-producing injuries that may be caused by dehydration [11]. Proper sleep and recovery time are important as part of the healing process and will support the reduction of inflammation [11, 12]. Cryotherapy is a classification of techniques involving cold and can come in the form of ice packs, ice baths, ice massage, etc. [11, 13]. Active recovery techniques, such as low-intensity light exercises or simple movement, can increase blood flow to the areas of inflammation and help to flush the area and reduce inflammation. Massage and bodywork, done by a professional or the athlete themselves, have been shown to support increasing blood flow and the reduction in the inflammatory process [11]. These techniques, combined with a sound diet, may help to limit the extent of inflammation following exercise.

9.5 Conclusion

Inflammation is the process by which the body reacts to a stimulus by attempting to stop, eliminate, and recover from it. Stimuli can come in a variety of forms from an injury to chronic physical stressors. As stated, the inflammatory process is a standard part of the recovery of athletes, we are not looking to eliminate this but rather limit the inflammatory process to better allow the athlete to recover as quickly as possible. Nutritional strategies that involve reducing pro-inflammatory foods, increasing anti-inflammatory foods, and supplementation combined with some focused recovery techniques can assist the athlete in the control of the inflammatory process allowing them to recover more quickly from exercise and improve performance. As the control of inflammation is more difficult as we age these tools can have a particular importance for a nutritional professional working with older athletes.

References

1 Seaman DR. The diet-induced proinflammatory state: a cause of chronic pain and other degenerative diseases?. *J. Manipulative Physiol. Ther.* 2002;25(3):168–179. doi:10.1067/mmt.2002.122324
2 Christ A, Lauterbach M, Latz E. Western diet and the immune system: an inflammatory connection. *Immunity* 2019;51(5):794–811. doi:10.1016/j.immuni.2019.09.020
3 Carrillo JA, He Y, Li Y, et al. Integrated metabolomic and transcriptome analyses reveal finishing forage affects metabolic pathways related to beef

quality and animal welfare. *Sci. Rep.* 2016;6:25948. Published 2016 May 17. doi:10.1038/srep25948

4 Daley CA, Abbott A, Doyle PS, Nader GA, Larson S. A review of fatty acid profiles and antioxidant content in grass-fed and grain-fed beef. *Nutr. J.* 2010;9:10. Published 2010 Mar 10. doi:10.1186/1475-2891-9-10

5 Maleki SJ, Crespo JF, Cabanillas B. Anti-inflammatory effects of flavonoids. *Food Chem.* 2019;299:125124. doi:10.1016/j.foodchem.2019.125124

6 Haß U, Herpich C, Norman K. Anti-inflammatory diets and fatigue. *Nutrients.* 2019;11(10):2315. Published 2019 Sep 30. doi:10.3390/nu11102315

7 Ricker MA, Haas WC. Anti-inflammatory diet in clinical practice: a review. *Nutr. Clin. Pract.* 2017;32(3):318–325. doi:10.1177/0884533617700353

8 Rawson ES, Miles MP, Larson-Meyer DE. Dietary supplements for health, adaptation, and recovery in athletes. *Int. J. Sport Nutr. Exerc. Metab.* 2018;28(2):188–199. doi:10.1123/ijsnem.2017-0340

9 Tanabe Y, Fujii N, Suzuki K. Dietary supplementation for attenuating exercise-induced muscle damage and delayed-onset muscle soreness in humans. *Nutrients.* 2021;14(1):70. Published 2021 Dec 24. doi:10.3390/nu14010070

10 Li Y, Yao J, Han C, et al. Quercetin, inflammation and immunity. *Nutrients.* 2016;8(3):167. Published 2016 Mar 15. doi:10.3390/nu8030167

11 Barnett A. Using recovery modalities between training sessions in elite athletes: does it help?*Sports Med.* 2006;36(9):781–796. doi:10.2165/00007256-200636090-00005

12 Irwin MR. Sleep and inflammation: partners in sickness and in health. *Nat. Rev. Immunol.* 2019;19(11):702–715. doi:10.1038/s41577-019-0190-z

13 Kwiecien SY, McHugh MP. The cold truth: the role of cryotherapy in the treatment of injury and recovery from exercise. *Eur. J. Appl. Physiol.* 2021;121(8):2125–2142. doi:10.1007/s00421-021-04683-8

10

Supplementation

10.1 Introduction

Any discussion about sports nutrition, particularly when we're talking about masters' athletes, invariably brings about the topic of supplementation use. While supplementation can be extremely important for the performance of athletes, particularly masters' athletes, it is important that supplementation be used as a means of assisting the athlete in reaching a peak level of performance and not as the primary basis for their nutritional plan. Too often in the world of sports nutrition, supplementation is discussed as a nutritional plan in it of itself but not as the final touch on the overall strategy. Supplementation is not a good substitute for a sound nutritional plan. Fitness magazines and the internet are full of advertisements about supplements, which can confuse an athlete into thinking that supplements are the most essential element of the nutritional plan. It is because of this that it is essential for an athlete to have a solid diet plan in place prior to starting a supplementation regime. Sports nutritionists, not just the author of this book, prefer for their athletes to focus on a whole food approach to improving performance before they begin to look at supplementation. This is true for a variety of reasons. First, food in its whole form carries fewer risks of side effects that can be seen due to both the unlabeled additives found in some supplements as well as the risks of hypersupplementation of an individual nutrient. Let us look at caffeine, a prominent performance supplement as an example. The consumption of coffee as a means of getting a performance benefit is less risky than taking a caffeine pill. Part of this is simply the amount of caffeine per serving of coffee is less than the amount found in supplements and the amount of coffee needed for a toxic dose is less likely to be achieved than if consuming caffeine supplements alone. Additionally,

Sports Nutrition for Masters Athletes, First Edition. Peter G. Nickless.
© 2025 John Wiley & Sons, Inc. Published 2025 by John Wiley & Sons, Inc.

when we look at supplements, we often see a problem with the quality of the supplements. The Food and Drug Administration does not regulate supplementations the same way that it regulates pharmacological interventions. Unfortunately, this means that unless the nutritional practitioner or athlete is very specific about the supplements they choose and the sources of supplements they acquire, there is always a chance for adulteration or inaccurate dosage, amongst other quality control concerns. This alone makes supplementation less desirable, when compared to its whole food counterparts. This is not to say that I don't recommend supplements; in fact, I have yet to meet a high-level athlete who does not take at least one or two supplements at some point during their training. Supplement recommendations can be for a variety of reasons. Most of these are to target a specific outcome. Muscle building and recovery supplements are intended to target supplying the athlete with the building blocks of muscle so that they can recover from their exercise. Ergogenic supplements on the other hand are a classification that, if taken in a sufficient dose, will provide the athlete with a performance edge; this is less about trying to make sure the athlete gets enough of a nutrient but rather to take enough to get a performance benefit. Supplementation should also be targeted to the individual's athlete's need, the individual sport, and the individual athletes' goals. Supplement decisions need to have a targeted effect in mind for their use. Finally, there needs to be an evidence-based approach to supplementation. Supplement plans need to have a basis in research for their recommendation. There is quite a bit of misinformation regarding which supplements are going to benefit an athlete. A critical examination of supplementation with a focus on what they can realistically do for the athlete is essential. This chapter will examine the major classifications of supplements and the more common supplements in these groups. This is not a complete list of every available supplement, but will cover many of the more common supplements that will benefit a master's athlete.

10.2 Supplementation vs Whole Foods

There is a longstanding debate in the nutrition community as to whether whole foods are better than supplements and vice versa. In other words, should the athlete try to get all their nutrients through diet, or should they be looking for supplements? Opponents of supplementation point to the synergistic effects of foods that may be more difficult to replicate with synthetic supplements. In this view, supplements would be of lesser quality; for example, an orange contains many more nutrients than just vitamin C (energy, water, fiber, etc.). So, in the case of eating an orange vs supplementing with vitamin C, we can see that there is a clear benefit to the whole food vs the supplement. Additionally, due to poor regulation of the supplement industry, whole food may be more safe when compared to the potential for adulterated supplements. On the other side of the argument, the proponents of supplementation point to the variability of whole foods in trying to target nutrition. Two different oranges, for example, may contain completely different concentrations of vitamin C; this is not an issue with a supplement which, assuming it is of good quality, would always have the same active ingredients every dose. Additionally, when trying to get a larger dose of a specific nutrient, it may be too difficult to consume enough food in the diet without deviation from diet plan. Supplements, on the other hand, allow for a much larger dose of some of these nutrients with little deviation from the eating plan. Let us look at vitamin D supplementation vs whole food for someone who is deficient in vitamin D. This person may need a very large, sometimes pharmaceutical, dose of vitamin D to achieve homeostasis. This amount of vitamin D cannot be provided adequately in the diet alone making supplementation essential. Additionally, some nutrients are not as obtainable in the diet from whole foods, making supplements much more of a feasible option. As you can see, the answer is more complicated than the question. For most macro- and micronutrients a whole food diet may be used to supply the athlete with all of the nutrients they will need for performance and recovery. That being said if the athlete is looking for larger dosages of some nutrients or they are not eating a diet rich in all nutrients supplementation may be an easier way for them to get the nutrients they need. If the athlete is looking to add the benefits from some of the more proprietary blends of nutrients then supplementation is a better option when compared to whole foods. On that note, if the athlete is looking to incorporate more herbs into their diet, it may be easier for them to acquire the herbs needed in a therapeutic volume through supplementation. One important consideration is supplement quality and adulteration in order to get the most benefit from the supplements, compared to whole food, they must be using a supplement of the highest quality. Additionally, since the adulteration of supplements is a concern for drug-tested athletes a whole food diet would be a better option for those who cannot source quality supplements.

10.3 Muscle and Tissue Repair and Growth

This category of supplements relates to those that are used by athletes to promote muscle repair and growth. It is through these supplements that athletes seek to provide the nutrients needed to promote recovery and growth following exercise. Often these nutrients are supplemented to the degree that exceeds what they get from their diet alone. These supplements are often used by bodybuilders and strength dependent athletes but have applications for all athletes. Bodybuilding and weight-dependent athletes may choose these supplements as they try to limit their caloric intake of whole foods while providing the nutrients needed directly. Additionally, for sports like bodybuilding, the consumption of some of these supplements may exceed the amount of food they could comfortably eat and still perform their athletic activities. Regardless of the reason, when an athlete consumes these nutrients, they are used to promote tissue repair and growth.

10.3.1 Protein Powders

Protein powders are among the top-selling sports supplements on the market today. Pages and pages of advertising in fitness and bodybuilding magazines have been devoted to the promotion of protein powders as a means of maximizing muscle repair and growth. This supplement, from a functional perspective, is the easiest to explain as a protein powder provides the athlete with the macronutrient protein with a small amount of other macronutrients. The goal of Protein powders is to replace some of the daily requirements for protein, as discussed in Chapter 4, with a powdered version that typically is ingested as a shake, although protein powder could be used in other recipes. There are differences in the type of protein, the source, and some potential additives in the form of added supplements, but at their core protein powders remain a basic supplement with little to no ambiguity. The International Olympic Committee (IOC) came out with a paper where they listed the top supplements that they recommended based on all available evidence collected over several years. The research was evaluated and discussed with a committee of renowned sports nutritionists. With all the evidence that surrounds protein and the importance of protein in the diet, specifically the role of protein in muscle and tissue repair, one would think that protein would have at least been on the list as a major, if not the top supplement, recommended for its ergogenic benefits. Yet protein does not make this list, but rather is listed as a functional food [1]. Protein is not noted as an ergogenic aid by the committee. This is not because the International Olympic Committee did not believe that protein was an important nutrient in the diet or that its supplementation would not benefit performance, but rather that supplemental protein was not needed in such an abundant quantity that it could not be obtained from food alone. A protein supplement is more as a convenience option to ensure adequate intake, particularly when eating whole food protein is not an option. If we were to look at a simple case example of an athlete, this athlete needs 1.4 g of protein per kilogram of body weight, as determined by the formulae related to protein needs for athletes. On a 100-kg frame, in this case, we see an athlete who only needs 140 g of protein. Now. If we were to look at the amount of protein in specific foods, we would see that one ounce of chicken contains approximately 7 g of protein. This would mean this 100-kg athlete only needs 20 oz of chicken per day in order to satisfy all of their protein requirements. While it may seem that 20 oz or 1 1/4 lbs. of chicken is a lot of chicken to consume over the course of a day. It's not an inordinate amount for a 100-kg individual. It would equate to little more than three 6 oz chicken breasts daily. Keep in mind that this amount would only need to be consumed if chicken was the only protein source the athlete chose. This is an unlikely scenario and foods such as eggs, milk, other meats, nuts etc., all make up the collective protein intake for an athlete during the course of a day. So it is, therefore, understandable that the International Olympic Committee intimate an athlete can get enough protein from their diet that they do not need to focus primarily on supplementation but rather to use it if the protein needs are not met by diet alone. That being said, there are a few rationales for increased protein quantities. Specifically, the International Society of Sports Nutritionists (ISSN) notes the need for increased protein depends on the type of sport and the goal of the athlete. The ISSN notes that amounts of protein as high as 4 g/kg of body weight are associated with improvements in body composition [2]. Additionally, the need for protein and the absorption of protein is not the same for older athletes when compared to younger athletes. This increases the requirements for protein in older athletes. Finally, some athletes simply do not want to, or have time to, cook and eat that much food during the course of a bust schedule. The athlete may not want to eat that much protein, either for personal preference or due to digestive issues or time constraints. Therefore, protein supplementation is one of the most common supplements ingested by athletes of all ages and is an important consideration for older athletes. When choosing a protein supplement, we must take into account the type and quality of the protein being used. As we stated in Chapter 4, not all protein sources contain identical amino acids or absorption rates. Therefore not all protein supplements carry the same efficacy for athletes.

In Chapter 4, the essentiality of protein was discussed as was the topic of amino acid completeness scores. The digestible, indispensable amino acid score (DIAAS) and various methods of assessing protein quality were explored in detail. The takeaway from this information is that if we are choosing to supplement the diet with protein then, just like when consuming protein, we need to take into account assessments like the digestible indispensable amino acid score and the overall completeness of the protein. The digestible indispensable amino acid scores of various proteins is different from the amino acid score or other measure in that it includes the digestibility by the distal ilium of protein. The higher the DIAAS score, the better the absorption and the potential for assimilation of the protein into muscular tissue. Therefore, it would be important to pick a protein with the highest DIAAS that the athlete feels comfortable consuming.

Another important consideration, in addition to the digestibility of a protein, is the speed at which the protein is digested. Take a look at the chart below, for example, which shows the absorption rates of different proteins. Notice, for example, that egg, or cow's milk-based proteins are absorbed slowly, whereas whey protein is absorbed more quickly. This is particularly true of whey hydrolysate protein due to its purity [3]. The absorption rate of the individual proteins should be taken into account when discussing the timing of protein consumption, for example, if we're looking to stave off catabolism and recover from exercise while we sleep, the athlete would want a slower digesting protein such as casein. On the other hand, if we're looking for a faster digesting protein for the time period immediately following a workout, then a whey protein, either concentrate or hydrolysate would be a more obvious selection. This brings us to the topic of targeting supplementation to a specific objective. The supplement suggested should always match a specific targeted outcome, typically in relation to the athlete's performance goal. In this manner, we can appropriately target the protein taken to the time period in which it is being ingested (Figure 10.1).

Another point for consideration when it comes to protein supplementation is the form of the supplement being consumed. Protein form refers to the level of purity or processing for the protein. Some proteins come in a more pure form, like an isolate, vs a less pure version such as a concentrate. There are also forms of protein that have added enzymes or are partially digested which can have an impact on protein assimilation. Whey concentrate, for example, is the most basic form of a whey protein supplement, but it can contain as low as 20% whey protein. The remainder of the serving being a combination of fillers. In this case, an athlete may need to ingest more of the supplement to get the desired effect. This can be compared to a whey isolate protein which can contain no less than a minimum of 90% whey protein [4]. Comparing whey isolate to a concentrate there is a larger percentage of the serving that actually

Egg	1.4 g/h
Pea	3.4 g/h
Milk	3.5 g/h
Casein	6.1 g/h
Whey	8–10 g/h

Figure 10.1 Protein absorption rates.

can be used to satisfy the performance objectives of taking the supplement in the first place. Looking at a whey isolate protein compared that to a hydrolysate protein, which is going to be not only pure but a partially digested protein, we see a much more high-quality protein. Unfortunately, with increases in quality, there will come an increase in price. Which for many athletes is an important consideration. In the ideal scenario, the athlete will be consuming the purest form of the supplement with a form that is most easily digestible, but financial considerations, and occasionally, the availability of the products can make athletes choose a less-desirable form for supplements.

We have discussed many of the relevant factors in relation to protein supplement consumption as a nutrient, but another important factor is the personal preference of the athlete. As mentioned earlier, there are a variety of reasons why an athlete may choose supplementation over food. For example, a vegetarian athlete may choose to get the majority of the protein in their diet from supplementation due to their desire to avoid animal protein. If a vegetarian athlete is in need of 160 g of protein, it is easier if a large portion of this comes from a plant based protein supplement rather than from vegetables alone. Unfortunately, some of the considerations that differentiate one protein source from another often have to do with the type of protein and amino acid makeup. Specifically in this case, some of the best protein powder supplements in terms of digestibility, absorption, etc. are animal-based. On a purely objective data-informed basis, it would seem that many protein powder supplements made from plant-based proteins are less desirable for athletes on the whole. This will become even more important when looking at methionine and lysine [5, 6]. Therefore, the type of protein, for example, whey, pea, casein, etc., used for supplementation has to include athlete preference factored in with the quality of the protein. Taste is also an important consideration related to athlete preference. The best protein is the protein that an athlete will actually consume and the better a protein tastes yet still meets the nutritional needs of the athlete, the better the protein for that athlete (to an extent).

10.3.2 Amino Acid Supplementation

Proteins are made up of amino acids joined together with peptide bonds. It stands to reason, therefore, that if the athletes are meeting their daily protein needs, then they are highly likely they are getting the full complement of amino acids. However, amino acid supplementation has come into and out of vogue for athletes for many years. Old bodybuilding magazines from the 60s were promoting amino acid supplements for athletes for muscle growth and recovery. Proponents point to the positive association between amino acid supplementation and muscle repair and growth. Opponents feel that targeted amino acid supplementation is unnecessary for athletes who are consuming enough protein to meet their requirements. In a few ways, both arguments carry validity at the same time. First, an athlete who is consuming protein that either meets or exceeds their individual protein requirements likely will be getting an appropriate amount of amino acids, if the protein is of sufficient quality and completeness. Second, there is minimal performance benefit to the over consumption of individual amino acids for athletes who are consuming their protein needs for the replenishment and growth. On the other hand, the physically stressful nature of many athletes' lives, physically, can render specific amino acids conditionally essential meaning that the need for specific amino acids may possibly be fluid depending on athlete presentation. Additionally, an athlete who is consuming a plant-based diet or who consumes most of their protein from less complete or digestible sources may have the need to ensure they meet their needs by considering dietary supplementation [7]. Many plant-based proteins are deficient in some amino acids such as methionine and lysine. To optimize performance these amino acids need to be gotten in some form. Finally, as many athletes participate in weight-dependent sports, there is often a tendency for athletes to restrict calories as part of a diet. While it is not only possible, but preferable for an athlete to diet and still meet the amino acid needs, at times, an athlete who is dieting or cutting weight may need to consider amino acid supplementation to ensure meeting their dietary needs. This necessitates a deeper look into amino acid supplementation.

10.3.3 Branched Chain Amino Acids

Although all of the essential amino acids are important for everyone in general and athletes in particular, the branched chain amino acids, lysine, leucine, isoleucine, and valine carry the greatest potential benefit for the competitive athlete. These specific amino acids have a more direct impact on athletic performance and should be considered to be taken as a supplement. These amino acids, not only participate in a variety of functional reactions related to physical performance, they are particularly beneficial for athletes who are cutting weight or dieting. In particular, it can help to provide the athlete with improved muscle growth, reduce fatigue and soreness, prevent muscle wasting, and energy to fuel performance [8]. The benefits of branched chained amino acids on older athletes for the aforementioned reasons as well as for the potential impact in mitigating some neurological impacts of aging, cannot be understated.

10.3.4 Branched Chain Amino Acids vs Essential Amino Acids

There is a running debate in the popular culture of the sports nutrition world as to whether it is better for the athlete, who chooses amino acid supplementation, to supplement with only branched chain amino acids or with all of the essential amino acids. This, of course, first requires an evaluation of the diet and if there is a need for supplementing amino acids at all. On one side of the debate, we see the argument that since all of the branched chain amino acids are all part of the essential amino acid classification, then any supplement with all essential amino acids will automatically include all the branched chain amino acids. Proponents of this school of thought feel that supplementation should be focused on the essential amino acids entirely, as these are needed from the diet for recovery and growth and will include all amino acids needed. On the other side of the argument, is the thought that branched chain amino acids are said to carry more of a direct impact on athletic performance and are needed in larger abundance for athletes compared to what would be found in essential amino acid supplements. This school of thought would support the use branched chain amino acid supplements as more focused on the needs of the athlete. To supplement the diet with all the essential amino acids does provide the athlete with all the branched chain amino acids but not necessarily in the quantity needed for optimal performance. Taking enough of an essential amino acid supplement to meet this need could lead to a need to an excess in the amount of some of the essential amino acids taken to support the branched chain amino acid needs. This would lead to the potential overconsumption of other essential amino acids that may not be needed in the same quantity. A third argument has come out recently that supports supplementation with both essential and branched chain amino acids as this will ensure the athlete meets their branched chain amino acid needs as well as their essential amino acid needs with less overconsumption [9, 10]. This third option or a version of it is intriguing as there are some benefits to an essential amino acid supplementation to athletic performance, yet as we will see some amino acids can have benefits if taken in larger does, such as leucine. This argument is of course predicated on the need for essential amino acid supplementation at all. As stated previously, most athlete will meet their essential amino acid needs through a well-designed diet alone and for them targeted individual amino acid supplementation may be a good option. For those on strict diets that may limit the essential amino acids (vegetarians, aggressive weight cuts, etc.), this combined strategy may provide the best means of ensuring maximal performance and recovery with a minimum of overconsumption of nutrients.

10.3.5 Leucine

Leucine is one of the four branched chain amino acids. Leucine has the specific potential to have a tremendous impact on sports performance. Recent research into the role of the amino acid leucine as a supplement for the promotion of muscle protein synthesis has demonstrated the potential to substantially impact athletes. Leucine has been shown in the research to stimulate muscle protein synthesis for athletes and non-athletes alike. Leucine has been used in the clinical setting as 6 g of leucine has been shown to reduce the muscle wasting seen in patients who have been diagnosed with sarcopenia. Part of the reason why whey is such an effective protein source for muscle building is that it has a significant dose of leucine per serving. This amount of leucine is more than is seen with many other protein sources, including some of the plant-based sources. This would indicate that there is some value in considering supplementation with leucine for certain athletes. This, of course, is not needed if the athlete is consuming enough leucine through their own dietary protein intake. A vegetarian athlete may consider leucine supplementation if their dietary protein sources do not contain enough leucine or they do not supplement with a leucine-rich protein. The same can be said for dieting athletes as the muscle protein synthesis effects of leucine may counteract any catabolism and muscle loss seen during lowered caloric intake. As we talk about the impact of sarcopenia as it relates to older athletes, the need for muscle protein synthesis should be paramount. It would be for this reason that leucine should be on any nutritional practitioner or coach's list of strongly recommended supplements for older athletes [11–14]. There is a strong evidentiary base to support the use of leucine for master's level athletes. While the impact of leucine supplementation on performance has not been studied in as much detail as some other nutrients, there is ample evidence to support the use of leucine to support post-exercise recovery and to prevent sarcopenia and muscle wasting in older adults who may not be getting enough from their diet. While leucine may not directly improve performance, it does appear to support athletes and indirectly have an impact on performance through enhanced recovery.

10.3.6 Ornithine

Ornithine is a nonessential amino acid that is associated with the regulation of various metabolic processes in the body. Working together with arginine and citrulline ornithine is part of the urea cycle, assisting the body in the removal of ammonia. Ammonia buildup can be a concern following intense cardiovascular workouts. This would mean that ornithine could benefit endurance athletes. Ornithine can also be involved in arginine production. Unlike other amino acids, ornithine does not make protein but is involved in processes associated with cell growth proliferation and proline production, which is associated with collagen synthesis, indicating that ornithine can have a role in supporting both the aerobic and anaerobic athlete. Ornithine has been associated with increasing the production of growth hormone in athletes. The impact of this has the potential to support the master's athlete to recover from exercise and improve their performance. There is some debate as to the effects of amino acid production on growth hormone production for strength athletes [15–18].

10.3.7 Glutamine

Glutamine is an amino acid, typically classified as non-essential, meaning the athlete does not typically need to get it in their diet but can become essential based on increased demand. This increase in demand for glutamine can come in many forms but is quite often the case with the stresses of high-intensity athletic activities. Glutamine has a few uses for the athlete. First of all, glutamine has a role in regulating the immune system and can help with support in fighting the inflammatory response. Glutamine can also be important for cell proliferation, energy production, energy storage, and for helping to regulate acid–base balance. These effects can have strong impacts for athletes as they can be associated with immune support and the reduction of fatigue and be considered effective as an ergogenic aid particularly for endurance athletes. Evaluation of glutamine has demonstrated research support for its role in regulating acid–base balance, energy production, and glycogen synthesis. The extent to which this can directly impact performance remains to be seen at this time, however as some research has shown the benefits of glutamine are more from the correction of deficiencies rather than supplementing beyond requirements. As a nonessential amino acid, the supplementation of glutamine for most causal athletes and those eating a well-balanced diet is not necessary. Athletes who are in a caloric deficit, participating in high-intensity sports, or participating in long-duration endurance sports like distance running and triathlons may find that they are at a greater risk of glutamine deficiency. Glutamine is attained through the diet from meats like beef chicken, fish, and eggs, as well as some legumes, tofu, and dairy. As a supplement Glutamine can be taken in in powder or pill form and is often added to protein powders. Glutamine should be taken within two hours of exercise completion to replace any loss during exercise and support recovery. Dosages of glutamine of up to 0.65 g/kg of body weight have been tolerated without negative effects [19–23].

10.3.8 Beta-alanine

Beta-alanine is the beta form of the non-essential amino acid alanine. It is referred as beta-alanine due to the attachment of the amino group being located on the second carbon from the carboxylate group or the beta carbon rather than the more typical alpha carbon. This amino acid is precursor to the synthesis of carnosine, which acts as a buffer in the muscles, from acidic buildup during anaerobic activities. Although beta-alanine is usually ingested in supplement form, alanine is typically produced in the liver and derived from animal foods eaten in the diet. Beta-alanine is an important and limiting ingredient in the production of carnosine. The effects of buffering of carnosine in the muscles carry the effects of reducing the acidity produced during high-intensity exercise. Accordingly, the effect of beta-alanine is that it can decrease the time to fatigue for high-intensity exercises, allowing for increased exercise intensity for athletes. The impacts of beta-alanine have been demonstrated primarily short-duration high-intensity activities, typically in the one to four minute range. Dosages of beta-alanine that have been shown to be effective have been in the 0.8–1.6 mg range every four hours up to approximately 4–6 mg daily. A negative side effect that has been noted with large doses of beta-alanine includes a sensation of tingling throughout the body. This sensation can be uncomfortable for many, but splitting the dosage into smaller amounts every four hours can minimize this feeling with no negative impact on the effectiveness of the supplement [24–27].

10.4 Carbohydrate Powders and Gels

As has been discussed in Chapter 4, carbohydrates are a major provider of the energy needed to fuel athletic performance. Although the extent to which they are used depends much on the sport being contested and the intensity of the activity, most athletic performance nutrition strategies will end up consisting of dietary carbohydrates. A well-designed nutritional plan remains the most efficient method of adding carbohydrates to the diet. Despite this, there are times when the supplemental forms of carbohydrates may be the preferred choice for an athlete. This may be due to convenience or even personal preference. For example, an athlete competing or training for an event may choose to add a carbohydrate powder to their drinks for intra-workout nutrition rather than eating a bagel during a football game. In this case, the athlete will need a fast-acting source of carbohydrates that can fuel continued exercise at a time when stopping to consume carbohydrates may not be the most convenient option, or even allowed by the sport. Carbohydrates can also be useful for the rapid replenishment of glycogen stores following a workout, or for the athlete looking to add calories to their diet as they are trying to gain weight. There are several carbohydrate options, each with some strengths and drawbacks. Dextrose and maltodextrin are the most common carbohydrate supplements used by athletes. Dextrose is a form of sugar that comes from corn or wheat and is very similar to glucose. This would have a rapid digestion and is readily available to be used by the athlete for energy. Maltodextrin is a polysaccharide so not as rapidly digested or sweet as dextrose, but it still can be digested rapidly [28]. These carbohydrate examples share the benefits of easy digestibility with a fast impact on performance. One potential drawback to these powders is the speed with which they can be digested and the potential for this to rapidly elevate blood sugar. This is a problem arising from the ingestion of such a fast-digesting carbohydrate, that is not as commonly seen in a well-designed whole food plan. This can be a benefit to an athlete during a competition but problematic at other times, specifically as it relates to long-term insulin control. It is for this reason that carbohydrate powders should be primarily consumed as part of an intra-workout nutrition plans and are not ideal for use outside of athletic events due to their impact on blood sugar. Another potential use for carbohydrate powders is that they provide the potential for the easy addition of calories to the diet. This is not needed for most athletes, but for athletes looking to put on weight who are unable to eat enough calories to achieve this may find benefit in a carbohydrate powder. Some bodybuilding nutritional plans call for a high amount of carbohydrates at times; the use of a carbohydrate powder can provide these carbohydrates in situations where the athlete is looking to add them to their diet quickly and easily. An athlete in this situation would see the benefits of adding 50–100 g of carbohydrates daily, ideally post-workout, to increase their total caloric intake by 200–400 calories.

Carbohydrate gels like carbohydrate powders provide a quick method for an athlete to ingest carbohydrates during exercise as a quick method of fueling performance and for refilling glycogen stores. Packaged in a quick "easy-to-open" pouch, these gels provide a significant portion of carbohydrate, typically in the forms that are quick to digest like maltodextrin or fructose. Although carbohydrates ingested immediately before or after workouts are beneficial for an athlete, the use of prepackaged gels tends to be associated with, and are best suited for, intra-workout nutrition. Some athletes will note that the sweetness of the gels can sometimes make them more difficult to stomach and, accordingly, are not the preferred choice for all athletes. These gels are best suited for endurance-based sports with a duration of over one hour which will typically require an intra-workout nutrition plan. These carbohydrate replacements have minimal value for athletes competing in sports of a shorter duration, as they often can use more traditional carbohydrate sources pre and post-workout and rarely need to refeed during a workout.

Recent studies have suggested that the commercially prepared carbohydrate gels do not have an increased value for energy replenishment when compared to pure honey or mashed potatoes. These two items are able to provide the athlete with the quick access energy needed for performance but at either a decreased cost or, in the case of mashed potatoes, more palatable saltier flavor. The sources of fast acting carbohydrates could be considered for intra-workout nutrition and can be used as per athlete preference. Some carbohydrate gels contain added micronutrients or other ingredients targeted to improve performance. One example here is caffeine, which can be added to gels to improve alertness, blood flow, and overall performance. Care must be taken to ensure the athlete is aware of any added ingredients and the potential risks they may impose (such as a caffeine overdose, for example). Additionally, there is a debate on whether the athlete should be consuming whole foods vs supplements for intra-workout nutrition. There are several points to consider. First, supplements are more convenient for many athletes. The value of whole food cannot be understated, but when targeting specific nutrients, it may be easiest to select pre-prepared targeted gels and powers (chews and jelly beans are available as well). Second, supplemental carbohydrates may be easier on the athlete's digestive system, while this may not be true for every athlete, some may find eating during an event to be a bit taxing on the digestive system. Finally, there is a question on the impact of a whole food choice on performance. This will not be a factor in every sport, but eating while actively competing may not be as beneficial to performance as quickly ingesting a carbohydrate-containing drink or gel. Looking at the example of a gel vs mashed potatoes, it may be a bit easier for a runner to quickly ingest a gel, when compared to mashed potatoes, while maintaining their pace [29, 30]. In the end, the use of gels, powders, or whole foods will always have the athlete's preference as a key factor. In all cases if two products are comparable in potential performance benefit, then athlete preference should be the top concern.

10.5 Vitamins and Minerals

The topic of vitamins and minerals, and their effects on performance have been discussed in Chapter 5. Rather than discussing them individually this section will discuss the use of a multivitamin supplement specifically.

The topic of a multivitamin for use by athletes is an interesting one. On one hand, we know that many micronutrients have important roles in energy production and recovery from exercise, making them essential for both health and performance. On the other hand, there have been many studies that have demonstrated that there is no significant improvement in sports performance for athletes who have taken a multivitamin in the absence of a deficiency. This would lead to the common argument that a multivitamin is not needed and is often excreted in the urine having done nothing for the athlete. The phrase "expensive urine" is often used to describe multivitamin use. Of course, this entire argument is predicated on the idea that an athlete is eating a diet rich in all micronutrients needed, even including accounting for the increased needs seen by athletes due to their increased physical activity. It is entirely possible for an athlete to get all of their micronutrient requirements from the diet but this may not be happening in reality. First of all, the athlete may be eating a limited diet, choosing to focus their calories on macronutrient needs for performance which could lead to micronutrient deficiencies. This is common for athletes who need to restrict food choices to accommodate macronutrient needs, for example. Additionally, athletes who are in some sports may see their need for micronutrients increases more than others, either due to the sport itself or other factors such as severe sweating, age, sex, etc. If the athlete does not take this into account in their diet, they may end up with a micronutrient deficiency. Even if the deficiency does not rise to the level of a health concern, it is possible for the athlete to be deficient enough to impair their performance. Athletes in weight-dependent sports may find their limited caloric intake can coincide with a decrease in micronutrient consumption, and as many macronutrients are involved in metabolic processes, an athlete eating more may have an increased need they may not be accounting for. Finally, older athletes will have an increased need for some micronutrients, calcium, and vitamin D, for example, and this must be accounted for in the diet to avoid deficiencies. For these reasons, I feel that the benefits of a multivitamin to an athlete involve the assurance that the athlete is meeting their micronutrient needs regardless of their specific diet. In this case, a multivitamin is not improving performance but acting as insurance in case the athlete's diet is deficient for some reason. There has also been some evidence to suggest the benefits of multivitamins on cognitive function for older adults. The author recommends all older athletes consider taking a multivitamin daily, unless they are doing a frequent dietary analysis and changing their diet to accommodate any deficiencies. Care must be taken to purchase a multivitamin from a high-quality company to both ensure the ingredients are as advertised and there is nothing in the multivitamin that should not be there [31–34].

10.6 Oxidative Stress

Oxidative stress is a term that describes what happens when the production of free radicals is greater than the availability of the antioxidants needed to reduce their effects. Free radicals are produced as a result of many biochemical reactions in the body. One example would be the production of ATP for use as energy, which will produce free radicals as a byproduct. Additionally, exposure to environmental pollutants, cigarette smoking, or radiation can all lead to increased free radical production as can the physical stresses of exercise. In a homeostatic state, these free radicals are counterbalanced by the production or ingestion of antioxidants, which can lend electrons to balance out the free radicals. If there is an imbalance caused by either excess production of free radicals or too few antioxidants, there will be health-related issues. The problem with an imbalanced state is that the elevations of circulating free radicals can, among other things, lead to performance and recovery decline, speed up some aspects of aging, and suppress immunity, making the individual more prone to illness and injury. This places an increased importance on the athlete maintaining a homeostatic balance between their oxidative stresses and their antioxidant defenses [35, 36]. While a diet that includes antioxidant-rich sources remains an ideal means of achieving this balance, supplementation of antioxidants is a big part of many athletes' regimes.

10.6.1 *N*-Acetylcysteine

N-acetylcysteine (NAC) is a supplement used to support a few biochemical processes. NAC is derived from the amino acid cysteine. NAC has been marketed as both a supplement and as a pharmaceutical agent. As of the writing of this book, both uses are still available, but there have been some recent suggestions that supplemental use should be limited or discontinued. NAC can be converted to glutathione and accordingly, since glutathione is a powerful antioxidant, NAC has a very strong antioxidant role. This is a common supplement used for a variety of reasons among them NAC is an antioxidant, has anti-inflammatory uses, can enhance insulin sensitivity, and increased nitric oxide activity. As a pharmaceutical agent, there are quite a few uses. Chief among them is that NAC has been used to treat acetaminophen toxicity. As an antioxidant NAC supports the reduction of free radical as glutathione by scavenging reactive oxygen species. As an anti-inflammatory agent NAC works through its antioxidant capacity, which will suppress the production of NFkB. The impacts of NAC on acetaminophen toxicity relate to its pharmaceutical use, but as a drug, NAC can bind acetaminophen in the liver for excretion and can be beneficial. Research on the athletic benefits for older adults has been focused on the lower dosages used supplementally that can have both antioxidant and anti-inflammatory benefits. Additionally, the benefits of supplementation with NAC have been seen with both improvements in athletes with insulin sensitivity and increases in nitric oxide activity, which can improve oxygenation to tissues by improving blood circulation [37–40].

10.7 Hormone Balance and Cortisol Control

Cortisol is an important hormone that has the impact of controlling the stress response. It would be inaccurate and incorrect to say that we should be eliminating all cortisol from our lives, but the health implications of reducing cortisol levels in our bodies can be significant and widespread. Excess cortisol represents a significant problem for the general population, especially looking at the role of the inflammatory response. This is a problem for the general, as well as the athletic population for a variety of reasons. Physical and emotional stress are among the reasons for elevated cortisol production, and this can negatively impact the amount of testosterone produced by an individual. In the chart below, we look at the biochemical process by which cholesterol and other dietary and hormonal precursors are broken into a variety of outcomes. Now while the subject of biochemistry is beyond the scope of this book. It is important to note that 1,7 hydroxyprogesterone, which is a byproduct of the breakdown of cholesterol, can be converted to DHEA. DHEA can then be converted to androstenedione and testosterone. Androstenedione can be converted to testosterone or it can be converted to cortisol. Studies have demonstrated that when cortisol increases testosterone can decrease and vice versa [41, 42]. This is due in large part to limitations in substrate therefore. Some important things we should be considering when looking to minimize the effects of excess cortisol and maximize hormonal balance include how can the athlete control cortisol production and how can the athlete maximize hormonal balance through supplementation (Figure 10.2).

10.7.1 Dehydroepiandrostendione (DHEA)

DHEA is a hormone, which is produced in the body's adrenal glands. DHEA is a direct precursor to androstenedione as well as can be converted to either testosterone or estrogen. The benefit of this would be the increased production of testosterone for the potential improvement of athletic performance.

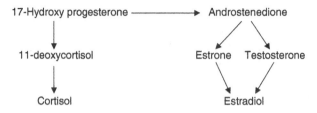

Figure 10.2 Biochemistry of cortisol synthesis.

Accordingly, it is through this relationship between DHEA and testosterone that we see the potential for increases in DHEA to benefit athletic performance. The implication being that the higher the levels of DHEA then the higher the levels of testosterone produced. Both exercise and caloric restriction can both increase the production of DHEA naturally, although caloric restriction may negatively impact performance in some sports. As people age, there is a natural reduction in DHEA production in the body, which may lead some athletes to supplement DHEA in an attempt to increase testosterone production. Studies have shown in older athletes that supplementation with DHEA has the capability of elevating the levels of free testosterone. This potential increase in testosterone is, understandably, important for masters athletes as the aging process naturally decreases testosterone levels. Supplemental forms of DHEA are available in both synthetic and natural forms, although a synthetic version will need a prescription for use. There is some suggestion that DHEA production can be increased through the consumption of foods such as wild yams although evidence does not support this. The effects of DHEA supplementation on muscle strength are inconclusive, with some studies demonstrating an increase in strength; others do not support this. Additional benefits of taking DHEA include its use in antiaging medicine due to its association with skin hydration, firmness, and reduced age spots. DHEA has been associated with reducing depression in those with low DHEA [43–47]. It is important to note that DHEA is on the list of substances banned by the WADA and that the use of DHEA for athletes is prohibited in many drug-tested organizations and should be avoided for athletes competing in these sports. This does not mean that there is no benefit for athletes, particularly master's athletes. DHEA is available for master's athletes to purchase, but due to the banned nature of DHEA, it should only be considered by athletes who do not plan to compete in tested events. Despite the research showing some positive effects, there is no scientific consensus on the use of DHEA. Males looking to enhance performance through testosterone increases may see some benefit loss as estrogen is also potentially increased with DHEA supplementation.

10.7.2 Tribulus Terrestris

Tribulus terrestris is a supplement derived from an herb that initially came from India. The primary use of tribulus terrestris for athletes is for the increase in testosterone production. One theorized reason for this is the ability of the saponins in the tribulus to increase the luteinizing hormone. The luteinizing hormone acts to increase testosterone production in the testis. A systematic review looking at the effects of tribulus terrestris on testosterone production was unable to substantiate the benefits of hormonal production [48, 49]. The same review noted that tribulus is considered safe with no demonstrated side effects.

10.7.3 Phosphatidylserine

Phosphatidylserine is a phospholipid that can help with the transmission of signals between the brain and nerve cells. There have been many health-related effects reported, including improvements in ADHD, Alzheimer's, depression, anxiety, and stress. The impact of phosphatidylserine on reducing stress is particularly important as stress leads to an increase in cortisol. It is through the reduction in stress that phosphatidylserine as the ability to indirectly increase testosterone production. In an athletic population, phosphatidylserine has been associated with the suppression of cortisol production and accordingly, increases in the conversion of 17-hydroxy progesterone into testosterone. This production of increased testosterone can result in a favorable hormonal balance for the athlete without having to take testosterone replacement therapy or DHEA [50–52]. Phosphatidylserine can be found in foods such as soy, white beans, egg yolks, chicken, and beef livers. Supplementation of phosphatidylserine is likely the best method to achieve the desired results. Studies have shown that while doses of up to 500 mg daily have been effective for cognitive function, 800 mg/day has been more effective for improved athletic performance. Some possible side effects from taking phosphatidyl serine include an upset stomach, gas, insomnia, and blood thinning.

As both Phosphatidylserine and DHEA will both potentially increase testosterone, why would one source be preferred to others? This would depend on the reason for the need to increase testosterone and other desired health effects. If the reason for the lowered testosterone has largely to do with overtraining and the stress response, then reducing cortisol may be the best option and phosphatidyl serine is the choice. If the concern is a lack of substrate from which testosterone can be made, then DHEA may be the best option. There is some research that both may work well for an athlete, but it is important to again reiterate that phosphatidylserine is not a banned substance, while DHEA is banned from drug-tested competition.

10.8 Inflammation Control

10.8.1 Fish Oil

Fish oil can be obtained by the athlete through supplementation or through the ingestion of fish and seafood in their diet. Fish oils derive their benefits from their Omega 3 fatty acid content in the form of eicosapentaenoic acid (EPA) and docosahexaenoic acid (DHA). These two fatty acids have important roles in the reduction of systemic inflammation and brain and nervous system health. High dosages of fish oil have been shown to be effective for lowering serum triglycerides, helping with fatty liver disease, and even reducing the incidence of flare-ups with rheumatoid arthritis. These essential fatty acids have slightly differing roles and therefore the mixture of each will determine the impact of the supplement on the athlete. Typically, we see a 2 : 1 ratio of EPA to DHA, which would lead to a product more likely to reduce the impact of inflammation for the athlete. A supplement like this is ideal for many athletes to use for everyday purposes. Higher amounts of DHA are used more for athletes who are looking for the impact on brain and nervous system health. These would include post-concussive athletes, younger athletes, and older athletes. So a masters athlete will want to make sure they are getting an appropriate amount of both EPA to control the inflammatory process and DHA to provide neurological support. Fish oil can be obtained from eating more fish such as Mackerel, Sardines, Tuna, and Salmon. The benefit of this is that fish oil comes from whole food sources that provide fatty acids as well as other nutrients that are important for performance, such as protein. I would not rely on eating fish alone as a primary source of fish oil if you are looking to get the maximal benefits as the amount of the oils per source may be too inconsistent. There may also be some legitimate concerns about seafood and mercury exposure, particularly with tuna. It would be for this reason that I would recommend eating fish that contains fish oil but supplementing additional fish oil. Fish oil supplements have been regarded as generally safe at dosages of up to 6 g for 12 weeks, although at dosages of over 3 g, there is an increased risk of bleeding. Most recommendations are for the athlete to use 1–2 g daily; masters athletes will want to get a higher amount of their fish oil to come from DHA than the typical 2 : 1 ratio. If one is consuming fish up to three times a week, supplementation beyond 1 g is not necessary; in fact, some studies suggest that supplementation beyond dietary intake has no benefit to performance [53–56].

10.8.2 Curcumin

Curcumin is a polyphenol that provides the pigment for the plant turmeric. This nutrient has been associated with both an anti-inflammatory as well as an antioxidant benefit that works by both neutralizing free radicals as an electron donor and through the reduction of pro-inflammatory cytokines. Curcumin has been used to treat a variety of inflammatory conditions due to its ability to inhibit inflammation. The primary benefit of curcumin for the athlete is the reduction of oxidative stress from exercise and to help with the reduction of exercise-induced inflammation thereby improving recovery from exercise. Curcumin has been shown to help reduce the inflammatory response of older adults with arthritis. Meta-analysis has demonstrated the safety and efficacy of curcumin in improving the symptoms of osteoarthritis. Additionally, curcumin has been associated with improving the post-exercise muscle soreness associated with athletics. Curcumin can be taken in whole food form by adding fresh turmeric as a spice to cooking, although many will use curcumin either as an oral supplemental form or as a topical cream. Curcumin is generally considered to be safe for consumption by athletes with performance benefits seen with dosages up to 500 mg [57–60].

10.8.3 Boswellia Serrata

Boswellia serrata, sometimes referred to simply as Boswellia, is a plant that has benefits as a potential anti-inflammatory agent. Boswellia is available in oral forms as well as in creams that can be applied topically. Boswellia is commonly used as an anti-inflammatory agent that can help with arthritis, asthma, and swelling or redness associated with inflammation as well as some other health-related benefits. Boswellia has been demonstrated to have an inhibitory effect on proinflammatory cytokines and can help to limit the inflammatory response. This has the benefit to the athlete of limiting the impact of the post exercise inflammatory response. Boswellia has been shown to be safe in typical dosages of up to 500 mg. Boswellia may have the potential to negatively interact with NSAIDs like aspirin and ibuprofen [61, 62].

10.8.4 Tart Cherry Juice

Tart cherry juice, as the name implies, is derived from the juice of tart cherries. Tart cherry juice as a food is known for its anti-inflammatory benefits. As a supplement, the juice is extracted and dried and typically sold as a powder or a pill, although a liquid supplement is available. The compounds in tart cherry include anthocyanins, flavonoids, and phenols. The compounds have anti-inflammatory and antioxidant benefits. This supplement has been shown to improve recovery, reduce inflammation, reduce muscle soreness, and improve sleep. Tart cherry juice is considered to be a safe supplement for use. Typically, the dosage of tart cherry juice is variable depending on the source, concentration and the form, liquid or powder, although 0.5–1 g/day is an approximate dosage for the powder form. Tart cherry juice is shown to be an effective means of helping to fight inflammation and accordingly is beneficial for master's athletes [63–65]. Although the same effects can be seen with eating tart cherries, the quantity required to see the benefits makes tart cherry supplementation more convenient.

10.8.5 Quercetin

Quercetin is derived from fruits and vegetables. This flavonoid is a powerful antioxidant that plays an important role in fighting inflammation. Quercetin is an oxygen donor that can neutralize free radicals and can inhibit the secretion of histamine, cytokines, and leukotrienes thus mitigating the inflammatory response. Due to its role in mitigating free radical damage and reducing inflammatory chemicals, quercetin has been associated with benefits for athletes as well as reducing the risks for some chronic diseases such as cardiovascular disease. This benefit is of increased significance when working with masters athletes as they have more issues with controlling inflammation and are at a greater risk with chronic noncommunicable diseases. These benefits carry a particular s Quercetin is generally considered to be safe as a supplement and the typical dosages are in the range of 500–1000 mg/day [66, 67]. Although food sources of the flavonoids exist, the quantity needed for the effects of the supplement form may make the supplement a more convenient means of getting them.

10.9 Ergogenic Supplements and Weight Loss

10.9.1 Creatine Monohydrate

Creatine monohydrate or simply creatine has become a "go-to" supplement in the sports nutrition world over the past three decades. There is good reason for this. This supplement has been used and researched substantially and even carries the support for its efficacy of the International Olympic Committee consensus statement on sports supplements. Although many forms of creatine exist on the market, the monohydrate form is the most studied and used version by athletes. Creatine is produced inside the body, through a process requiring the amino acids glycine, arginine, and methionine, as well as taken in its supplement form. The impact of creatine on athletic performance is related to the elevation of the body's internal creatine stores, which can result in a more rapid production of ATP for use to meet the energy requirements of the athlete. This allows an athlete to see performance benefits at higher training intensities. The combination of heavy resistance training and elevated creatine stores has been associated with an increase in the total maximal muscle strength and enhanced muscle mass of an athlete. Due to the energy systems used by anaerobic athletes, the effects of creatine supplementation are greater in those participating in activities that use the phosphagen energy system primarily. This is not to say that there is not a benefit to athletes competing in sports that extend into the glycolytic pathways either, particularly through the potential suppression of the lactate threshold. The combination of high carbohydrate diets with creatine supplementation has been shown to increase stored glycogen in muscles. Evidence supports the use of creatine supplementation can have a small benefit to body composition with older adults. Creatine supplementation has been noted to enhance the repair and recovery process, as well as aid neurological function. Creatine has been shown to help maintain muscle strength and prevent sarcopenia in older adults. Although there is generally strong support for creatine supplementation, it should be noted that not every athlete will respond to creatine supplementation in the same way or at all with a small percentage of non-responders or low responders. Creatine supplementation is body weight dependent and for most populations, a dosage of 0.1 g/kg body weight has shown to carry performance benefits with minimal side effects as creatine supplementation is generally considered to be safe [1, 68–70].

10.9.2 Sodium Bicarbonate

Sodium bicarbonate, known as sodium hydrogen carbonate or commonly as baking soda, is a common supplement taken by athletes for its effects as a buffering agent. Baking soda is very well known as a cleaning agent, but the ability to buffer a strong acid makes sodium bicarbonate a beneficial supplement for reducing the acidity in muscles produced by high-intensity exercise. Sodium bicarbonate has shown itself to be of most benefit to exercises that last in durations of 30 seconds up to 12 minutes, according to the International Society of Sports Medicine. This would mean that sodium bicarbonate has strong effects in high-intensity sports and endurance events such as cycling and running events. Dosages for sodium bicarbonate have been shown to be effective in the 0.2–0.4 g/kg range and recommendations are to either split this dose throughout the day or to take the total dosage no sooner than 180 minutes to the event. Side effects from sodium bicarbonate can include abdominal pain, nausea, diarrhea, bloating, and vomiting. These side effects do not affect every athlete the same way and tend to be dose-dependent, so an athlete should consider starting at a lower daily dosage or splitting the dosage throughout the day. Additionally, taking sodium bicarbonate with a high carbohydrate meal may reduce any abdominal side effects. Although usually found as a powder, sodium bicarbonate is available in an enteric-coated capsular formulation, which may reduce some of the potential side effects. Generally, the use of sodium bicarbonate is both safe and effective as a supplement to limit the impact of acid build-up in the muscles during high-intensity exercise [1, 71–73].

10.9.3 Caffeine

Caffeine is a commonly consumed stimulant that can be found as a naturally occurring ingredient in foods such as chocolate and in beverages like tea and coffee. Chemically, caffeine is known as 1,3,7-trimethylxanthine. Caffeine primarily acts on the central nervous system by blocking adenosine receptors, increasing the release of neurotransmitters such as dopamine, acetylcholine, and serotonin. Physically, caffeine is a nervous system stimulant that impacts increasing alertness and concentration and delaying fatigue. Caffeine impacts the functions of the nervous system, endocrine system, cardiovascular system, and muscular system. Caffeine has been shown to be effective in improving endurance performance times, reducing muscular fatigue from high-intensity exercise, and increasing maximal strength. Additionally, consumption of caffeine has the capability to increase the number of calories burned assisting with fat loss. Athletes find the consumption of caffeine beneficial for performance, but this impact is not uniform. A study examined the effects of caffeine on sports performance for subjects with different genetic variants and found that depending on the genetic subtype the effects of caffeine are different or even not effective. Additionally, regular caffeine users do not see the same benefits from caffeine use in performance compared to those who do not regularly consume caffeine. In relation to older athletes caffeine can be a very beneficial ergogenic aid, but care must be taken in this age group as there are many older athletes with comorbidities that may be impacted by caffeine consumption. Caffeine can raise both blood pressure and heart rate, and accordingly for those with cardiovascular problems, this may present an increase in health risk. Additionally, as older athletes have to pay more attention to hydration status when compared to younger athletes it is imperative that an older athlete who wants to use caffeine make sure to also monitor their hydration status to help mitigate this risk. Caffeine can also elevate the basal metabolic rate for individuals, which can have the effect of assisting the athlete to lose body weight and body fat. Caffeine has performance benefits for both endurance athletes as well as for strength athletes. Although the impacts of caffeine on sports performance are generally considered to be positive, some athletes can see little or even a negative effect of caffeine on their performance. The position of the International Society of Sports Nutrition supports the positive effects of caffeine on many, but not all athletes, particularly those competing in endurance events. Their support the positive effects of caffeine in the 3–6 mg/kg range (meaning a 100 kg athlete could consume 100–600 mg daily) with an increased risk of side effects above this amount. Individuals may find personal tolerances to caffeine to be different and accordingly should start at a smaller dosage to avoid any negative effects. Side effects of excess caffeine include increased heart rate, anxiety, dizziness, tremors, stomach pain, insomnia, and irritability. Additionally, excess caffeine can contribute to an increased risk of dehydration due to its role as a diuretic. Several medical conditions such as high blood pressure GERD and pregnancy have been noted as contraindications for caffeine consumption [74–79]. The amount of caffeine in each food or drink can vary greatly and each must be considered when making choices for consumption. A cup of coffee may have 100–150 mg per 8 oz serving but an energy drink can be significantly more. Many people choose to consume caffeine as part of a pre-workout supplement or as a single nutrient supplement. In a pre-workout supplement one must be careful of not only the caffeine content but also the content of other nutrients. Caffeine pills taken as a supplement typically contain about 200 mg per pill. This can provide a large amount of caffeine all at once. The benefit is that there is an ability to control the amount consumed and know exactly how much is consumed. The negative to this would be that it is much easier to overconsume and risk toxicity. If someone were to consume four 200 mg pills, they could do so all at once, but at 150 mg per 8 oz cup of coffee, they would need to consume over five cups to get that amount. This amount of coffee may be too much for one to consume and unlikely in the same short period. Caffeine can be an aid to sports performance, but care must be taken due to the potentially negative effects of overconsumption.

10.9.4 Nitric Oxide

Nitric oxide is a supplement that comes from various sources, including from beet juice. In fact, some recommend taking a beet juice supplement or consuming beet juice as a precursor to nitric oxide. Nitric oxide supplements contain ingredients that can be converted to nitric oxide such as arginine, citrulline, and beetroots. Nitric oxide is an important compound involved in several physiological processes. Nitric oxide has a few benefits for the athlete; it is a vasodilator that increases blood flow to bring oxygen and nutrients to the area. This can enhance energy and endurance. It is this vasodilatory effect that increases the pumped feeling that athletes feel after a workout. Nitric oxide can supply the blood vessels and have a potentially positive impact on cardiovascular health. Another benefit of nitric oxide is that it can support erectile function. There are not a lot of studies on the long-term effects of nitric oxide or its long-term safety. Typical dosages of nitric oxide are typically in the 3–6 g/day range [80, 81].

10.9.5 Chromium

Chromium is an essential trace mineral. Its essentiality means that it is required from the diet either from whole food or in supplement form. As a mineral, its functions include the support of carbohydrate, fat, and protein metabolism. Deficiencies in chromium can result in reduced insulin sensitivity, which can negatively impact blood glucose, weight loss, poor lipid blood profile, and peripheral neuropathy. Food sources of chromium include lentils, whole wheat bread, beef, eggs, chicken, etc. Athletes use chromium, typically in the form of chromium picolinate, as a means of supporting glucose sensitivity and assisting in fat metabolism, which can support fat burning. Chromium is also used to support the metabolism of BCAAs through enhanced transport of insulin into the muscles. Evidence for chromium use by athletes suggests chromium has a role in supporting decreased body fat in some participants, improving body composition and strength, with some studies suggesting increased aerobic performance with the use of chromium. Athletes will have a greater turnover of chromium compared to non-athletes, and accordingly, there is an increased need for chromium in an athlete's diet. The impacts of chromium picolinate on performance are not without debate, with some studies reporting no benefit on sports performance beyond supporting deficiency. This leads to the use of chromium as more about ensuring sufficient intake rather than an ergogenic aid. There is some concern that large dosages of chromium, as seen in supplementation, can have the potential to negatively impact the actions of some medicines [82–85].

10.9.6 Chitosan

Chitosan is a nutrient derived from chitin, which is what gives structure to the shells of shellfish, such as shrimp, crabs, and some mushrooms. Chitosan has a variety of purposes for food manufacturing but it is a commonly sold supplement used to help to promote weight loss. Chitosan's mechanism of action is to bind ingested fat and cholesterol, keeping it from being absorbed, resulting in weight loss and lowered serum cholesterol. Some studies do support the use of Chitosan as an adjunct to weight loss but not all studies support the effectiveness of chitosan for this purpose. There is also some evidence that chitosan can help modulate glycemic levels, assisting those with metabolic syndrome. This benefit can be particularly helpful for older athletes with difficulty controlling their blood sugar. Chitosan is generally considered to be safe as a supplement, although no ideal dosage has been identified [86–88].

10.9.7 Ephedrine

Ephedrine is a stimulant that works on the central nervous system to raise blood pressure, dilate blood vessels, and expand the lungs to improve breathing. All of these functions are associated with the sympathetic nervous system's fight-or-flight response. Medically, ephedrine is used as a decongestant and a treatment for low blood pressure as well as other breathing issues. Some of the side effects of ephedrine use include, but are not limited to, increased pulse, blood pressure, nervousness, anxiety, appetite, and weight loss. It is through the actions of ephedrine as a stimulant that it is used by athletes to increase performance. Research has shown that the increase in blood flow from the vasodilation mixed with the increase in oxygen from the bronchiole dilation that we see an increase in the impacts of aerobic-based activity. The impact of being a central nervous system stimulant has been shown to increase maximal strength in some studies. In addition to the ergogenic aid benefits seen with ephedrine, the increased metabolic activity seen from the stimulant effects, combined with the effects of a loss in appetite, show that ephedrine is used as an effective weight loss aid for some athletes. Overuse of ephedrine can be problematic, particularly for those with high blood pressure or any cardiac issue, making the use of ephedrine potentially deadly and any decision to use it should be discouraged. In the case of ephedrine, the potential for a negative outcome makes the risk outweigh the potential benefit. It is due to the potential for negative effects that ephedrine is on the WADA-banned substances list [89–91].

10.9.8 Pre-workout Supplementation

Pre-workout supplements are not as much a specific supplement as a classification of supplements, as such many of the ingredients have already been mentioned in this chapter. For example, caffeine, ephedrine, beta-alanine, BCAAs, nitric oxide, and creatine for example are common ingredients in pre-workout supplements. Additionally this classification can include ingredients that are not as well studied or may even be on the banned substances list. Often ingredients and amounts can be hidden from the consumer as part of a proprietary blend, which does not always need to be disclosed [92]. Many of the benefits of pre-workout supplements are similar to the ingredients they contain and include increased blood flow and pump, increased alertness, decreased fatigue during workouts, and enhanced recovery following workouts. Additionally, pre-workout supplements are central nervous system stimulants which, as discussed earlier, have been shown to improve performance in athletes [93]. These benefits are clear for the athlete, but they also have known negative effects such as potentially negative effects on blood pressure and pulse, increased risk of dehydration, and potential GI disturbances, among others [78]. This, of course, is not including any negative effects of banned substances that may be found in the product. Despite the benefits of many of the supplements commonly used on pre-workout formulations, the lack of transparency with proprietary ingredients, and the potential to contain substances banned by the WADA, their use is not recommended. This is not to say that a pre-workout supplement that contained a defined dosage of caffeine, creatine, beta-alanine, and BCAA would not be recommended for use, but rather the athlete should avoid any supplement without clearly defined ingredients.

10.10 Microbiome Support

Although it is often difficult for an athlete to see the connection between gastrointestinal health and athletic performance. The microbiome refers to the microorganisms that reside in the human body, the majority of which are in the gastrointestinal tract. The microbiome has important effects on the overall health of the athlete. The microbiome has impacts on areas such as the immune system, the endocrine system, gastrointestinal health, and even mental health. Although exercise has a positive association with a healthy microbiome, the physical stressors of heavy athletics, the lack of variation in the diet of the athletes, the impact of supplementation, and the effects of aging can lead to potential imbalances in the microbiome [94, 95]. With this in mind, it is important for an older athlete to focus on promoting health in their microbiome. This would include targeting dietary plans to those that promote a healthy microbiome such as reduced processed foods, reduced sugars, increased dietary fiber, and eating a diverse diet, particularly in terms of diversity of fruits and vegetables. In addition to this, there are some supplements that can be beneficial for the athlete to support their microbiome. Among these the most prominent would be probiotics and prebiotics.

10.10.1 Probiotics

Probiotic supplements are supplements aimed at promoting the health of the gut microbiome. They do this by providing live bacteria or yeasts in quantities that would be beneficial to a healthy microbiome. The microbiome is associated with many biochemical processes from controlling inflammation to having a role in proper digestive function. A healthy microbiome is possible through dietary changes, but it is with supplementation that we can see the impact of probiotics quicker. Part of the reason for this is the concentration of the live cultures in the supplement vs the food versions. As an athlete, there are many tangible benefits to a properly functioning microbiome as it will assist the athlete in controlling inflammation, assisting with recovery, supporting mental health, and supporting the digestive system which is required for optimal performance. These roles have a greater significance for master's athletes, who have often accumulated a lifetime of alterations to their microbiome. Probiotic supplements are generally considered to be safe for athletes. Dosages of probiotics are varied but range from 1 to 10 billion colon-forming units [96–98].

10.10.2 Prebiotic Supplements

Prebiotic supplements are supplements that contain undigestible fibers. These un-digestible fibers are fermented in the body and promote the growth of healthy bacteria. These have a different effect compared to probiotics in that prebiotics support the growth of healthy bacteria, whereas prebiotics provide the microbes directly. These both are beneficial when used in tandem. Prebiotic supplements are generally considered safe for use and dosages range from 5 to 10 g daily [98, 99].

10.11 Bone and Joint Support

10.11.1 Glucosamine

Glucosamine is an amino sugar found in the joints of the body and provides some of the building blocks of tendons, ligaments, cartilage, as well as synovial fluid. These roles are part of the repair and maintenance of the joints and demonstrate why glucosamine is often associated with joint health. This chemical can be ingested in the diet and is found in shellfish. Commonly glucosamine is taken in a supplemental form, as glucosamine sulfate, glucosamine hydrochloride, and *N*-acetyl glucosamine. Among these glucosamine sulfate is the most commonly known variety and is often seen combined with Chondroitin. Glucosamine is commonly taken for helping with osteoarthritis, joint pain, rheumatoid arthritis, and even multiple sclerosis. Among these uses, the evidence is strongest for the positive impact on glucosamine sulfate helping with relieving the pain and improving function for those with Osteoarthritis. There is no evidence that glucosamine will prevent osteoarthritis but rather provide support and help with symptoms for those suffering with osteoarthritis. As masters level, athletes are more likely to be suffering with these symptoms and reduced function, when compared to younger athletes, it would stand to reason that a glucosamine sulfate supplement should be considered for any older athlete, particularly those who are experiencing joint pain. Evidence suggests that oral supplementation is safe for daily use of up to 1500 mg for three years. Longer timeframes may be safe but have not been studied as extensively. There is the risk of some interactions with medication, for example, there has been some evidence that glucosamine may increase the effects of warfarin, used to slow blood clotting, which may lead to bleeding and bruising concerns. It is important that patients consult with their physician before taking supplements. Glucosamine is derived from shellfish and therefore some care should also be taken for those with a shellfish allergy [100–102].

10.11.2 Chondroitin

Chondroitin is a chemical found in the body as a component of cartilage. There are no major dietary sources for chondroitin, and it is usually ingested as a supplement in the form of chondroitin sulfate, commonly in conjunction with glucosamine, and derived commonly from shark and bovine cartilage. It is important to note that consumption of bone broth or shellfish can provide some chondroitin, but not as much as with supplementation. Chondroitin exerts its effects on cartilage by absorbing fluid into connective tissue, blocking some of the enzymes that break down cartilage, and providing the components that would be required to make new cartilage. Chondroitin is taken for the reduction of pain, swelling, and lost function associated with osteoarthritis. As with glucosamine, masters athletes with arthritis may find chondroitin to be an important addition to their supplement regime. While there is some dispute over the efficacy of chondroitin for the support of osteoarthritis, there are some studies that demonstrate a positive impact in the reduction of joint pain for those taking Chondroitin. Some studies show that chondroitin must be taken for a period, usually two to four months, before a reduction in symptoms is noted, although the effects have been shown to have a positive impact for up to three months after cessation of use. Effective dosages for chondroitin are 1200 mg daily, either as 400 mg 3×/day or 600 mg 2×/day. Chondroitin sulfate is considered a generally safe supplement, although some drug interactions have been noted, such as with anti-coagulants and NSAIDs, and therefore consultation with a physician is recommended before taking chondroitin [103, 104].

10.11.3 Methylsulfonylmethane

MSM is a naturally occurring form of sulfur that is found in some fruits, vegetables, grains, beer, coffee, and cow's milk. Commonly MSM is taken as a supplement and often combined with glucosamine and chondroitin. The common use for MSM is as an anti-inflammatory supplement, as an antioxidant, as a pain reliever for joint and muscle pain, and decreases in function due to osteoarthritis, among other, less-common use. Evidence supports its use for supporting athletes with osteoarthritis. The actions of MSM on supporting joints combined with the anti-inflammatory and antioxidant benefits would indicate that this supplement could be helpful for a master's athlete. MSM has been generally recognized as safe and well tolerated in dosages of up to 4000 mg daily. No major interactions have been noted with supplementation, although some mild side effects such as nausea, diarrhea, bloating, and stomach pain have been reported [105, 106].

10.12 Supplement Quality

A final word to consider when discussing supplementations for athletes in general, and older athletes in particular, is the importance of finding a good quality source of supplements. This is important for several reasons. First, there is the efficacy of the supplement; a higher quality supplement has more of a chance that it contains the amount of the ingredient that is listed on the label is actually in the product. This would mean that there is a greater chance that the athlete is getting the suggested dosages. Or conversely, if they are taking a poor-quality supplement there is the potential that the athlete is getting less of the active ingredient per serving than they wanted. A second reason for buying a good quality supplement is that there is less of a chance that there will be off-label ingredients, either as a filler or as an intentional addition. This carries a variety of impacts. An athlete who is taking a poor-quality supplement, for example, may be taking a variety of fillers that can have potential side effects that impact the health of the athlete. Regarding intentional off-label additions, the concern here is the impact on performance for a drug-tested athlete. Research has shown high percentages of supplements have been tainted or adulterated to include banned supplements. Unfortunately, many of the supplements that can be found on the shelves of many nutrition stores contain ingredients that are not listed on the label [107, 108]. Some of this adulteration can be done to substitute a cheaper ingredient for a more expensive ingredient. Another reason for the adulteration of supplements is the use of pharmacological agents and ergogenic aids that can carry health risks, as well as are not legal for use in most competitive sporting environments. The health implications of taking ergogenic aids or supplements that carry pharmacological agents are relatively well-known and should not be taken lightly. What is not discussed enough, though is the impact of these supplements on drug testing. It's not uncommon for older athletes to be competing in drug-tested sports. Some supplement companies will carry products that either inadvertently or intentionally contain banned substances or are produced alongside supplements that would be legal but still banned in sports but carry the risk of cross-contamination with other supplements. Drug testing cannot, unfortunately, tell whether the athlete meant to take an illegal substance intentionally or not and the athlete will be punished as if taking the substance was 100% intentional. Nobody who works with an athlete wants to be responsible for any negative repercussions to their health or their ability to compete due to failed drug testing. Therefore, it's extremely important that the athlete or practitioner find supplement sources that have been vetted for purity and quality. There are some agencies such as the NSF certified for sports programs. That seek to help athletes find supplements that have undergone voluntary testing for quality and purity. While not all of these voluntary certifications are trustworthy some, like NSF, can help an athlete to know that they have a supplement that should not cause a failure on a drug test and will contain the ingredients listed on the label. Even if the athlete is not competing in a drug-tested sport, it is still a good idea to seek out quality-controlled supplements, to minimize potentially negative health implications.

10.13 Conclusion

As stated, supplementation should not be the first choice for any practitioner or athlete looking to improve performance and recovery. A strong focused dietary plan needs to be the backbone of a performance strategy and supplementation should be used to finish out this strategy by accounting for any shortfalls and or providing performance benefits. Supplementation, when used, should be targeted to a specific goal so that the athlete may better achieve their desired outcome. This is going to be different than the goals of the athlete toward their overall performance or the goals of the athlete that were evaluated for determining macro and micronutrient load. By achieving their desired outcome, the author means, why are we supplementing this athlete? What are we trying to achieve with supplementation and what is the plan? For example, are we trying to help them build muscle tissue, in which case, we need to pick supplements targeted toward building muscle tissue? Are we trying to control inflammation? In which case we should pick supplements aimed at helping to control inflammation. It is very important that supplementation be used to help the athlete to achieve a specific end point or goal, and not just simply prescribed because many athletes utilize them. Common supplementation goals include but are not limited to the control of inflammation, the repair or building of tissue, support of the endocrine system, enhanced recovery from a sport or activity, or the restoration of gut health. In addition to being targeted to an overall performance goal, supplementation needs to be based on solid scientific data for efficacy. This chapter discusses many of the supplements used by athletes today but does not provide an exhaustive list. Care needs to be taken by the nutritional professional to keep up to date with the supplements that may impact their athlete's performance, the evidence for their use, and the risks associated with them. Used properly and for the right reason, supplementation can have a positive impact on helping the athlete maximize their capabilities.

References

1. Maughan RJ, Burke LM, Dvorak J, et al. IOC consensus statement: dietary supplements and the high-performance athlete. *Br. J. Sports Med.* 2018;52(7):439–455. doi:10.1136/bjsports-2018-099027
2. Jäger R, Kerksick CM, Campbell BI, et al. International Society of Sports Nutrition Position Stand: protein and exercise. *J. Int. Soc. Sports Nutr.* 2017;14:20. Published 2017 Jun 20. doi:10.1186/s12970-017-0177-8
3. Bilsborough S, Mann N. A review of issues of dietary protein intake in humans. *Int. J. Sport Nutr. Exerc. Metab.* 2006;16(2):129–152. doi:10.1123/ijsnem.16.2.129
4. Gorissen SHM, Crombag JJR, Senden JMG, et al. Protein content and amino acid composition of commercially available plant-based protein isolates. *Amino Acids* 2018;50(12):1685–1695. doi:10.1007/s00726-018-2640-5

5 Burke LM, Winter JA, Cameron-Smith D, Enslen M, Farnfield M, Decombaz J. Effect of intake of different dietary protein sources on plasma amino acid profiles at rest and after exercise. *Int. J. Sport Nutr. Exerc. Metab.* 2012;22(6):452–462. doi:10.1123/ijsnem.22.6.452

6 Ferrando AA, Wolfe RR, Hirsch KR, et al. International Society of Sports Nutrition Position Stand: effects of essential amino acid supplementation on exercise and performance. *J. Int. Soc. Sports Nutr.* 2023;20(1):2263409. doi:10.1080/15502783.2023.2263409

7 Shimomura Y, Kitaura Y. Physiological and pathological roles of branched-chain amino acids in the regulation of protein and energy metabolism and neurological functions. *Pharmacol. Res.* 2018;133:215–217. doi:10.1016/j.phrs.2018.05.014

8 Børsheim E, Bui QU, Tissier S, et al. Effect of amino acid supplementation on muscle mass, strength and physical function in elderly. *Clin. Nutr.* 2008;27(2):189–195. doi:10.1016/j.clnu.2008.01.001

9 Hulmi, JJ, Lockwood, CM, Stout, JR Effect of protein/essential amino acids and resistance training on skeletal muscle hypertrophy: a case for whey protein. *Nutr. Metab. (Lond).* 2010;7, 51. doi:10.1186/1743-7075-7-51

10 Martínez-Arnau FM, Fonfría-Vivas R, Buigues C, et al. Effects of Leucine administration in sarcopenia: a randomized and placebo-controlled Clinical Trial. *Nutrients.* 2020;12(4):932. Published 2020 Mar 27. doi:10.3390/nu12040932

11 Martínez-Arnau FM, Fonfría-Vivas R, Cauli O. Beneficial effects of leucine supplementation on criteria for sarcopenia: a systematic review. *Nutrients* 2019;11(10):2504. Published 2019 Oct 17. doi:10.3390/nu11102504

12 Martinho DV, Nobari H, Faria A, et al. Oral branched-chain amino acids supplementation in athletes: a systematic review. *Nutrients* 2022;14(19):4002. Published 2022 Sep 27. doi:10.3390/nu14194002

13 Oh GS, Lee JH, Byun K, Kim DI, Park KD. Effect of intake of leucine-rich protein supplement in parallel with resistance exercise on the body composition and function of healthy adults. *Nutrients* 2022;14(21):4501. Published 2022 Oct 26. doi:10.3390/nu14214501

14 Sivashanmugam M, Jaidev J, Umashankar V, Sulochana KN Ornithine and its role in metabolic diseases: an appraisal. *Biomed. Pharmacother.* 2017;86:185–194. doi:10.1016/j.biopha.2016.12.024

15 Zajac A, Poprzecki S, Zebrowska A, Chalimoniuk M, Langfort J. Arginine and ornithine supplementation increases growth hormone and insulin-like growth factor-1 serum levels after heavy-resistance exercise in strength-trained athletes. *J. Strength Cond. Res.* 2010;24(4):1082–1090. doi:10.1519/JSC.0b013e3181d321ff

16 Mikulski T, Dabrowski J, Hilgier W, Ziemba A, Krzeminski K. Effects of supplementation with branched chain amino acids and ornithine aspartate on plasma ammonia and central fatigue during exercise in healthy men. *Folia Neuropathol.* 2015;53(4):377–386. doi:10.5114/fn.2015.56552

17 Chromiak JA, Antonio J. Use of amino acids as growth hormone-releasing agents by athletes. *Nutrition.* 2002;18(7–8):657–661. doi:10.1016/s0899-9007(02)00807-9

18 Cruzat V, Macedo Rogero M, Noel Keane K, Curi R, Newsholme P. Glutamine: metabolism and immune function, supplementation and clinical translation. *Nutrients* 2018;10(11):1564. Published 2018 Oct 23. doi:10.3390/nu10111564

19 Coqueiro AY, Rogero MM, Tirapegui J. Glutamine as an anti-fatigue amino acid in sports nutrition. *Nutrients* 2019;11(4):863. Published 2019 Apr 17. doi:10.3390/nu11040863

20 Gleeson M. Dosing and efficacy of glutamine supplementation in human exercise and sport training. *J. Nutr.* 2008;138(10):2045S–2049S. doi:10.1093/jn/138.10.2045S

21 Holeček M Side effects of amino acid supplements. *Physiol. Res.* 2022;71(1):29–45. doi:10.33549/physiolres.934790

22 Ramezani Ahmadi A, Rayyani E, Bahreini M, Mansoori A. The effect of glutamine supplementation on athletic performance, body composition, and immune function: a systematic review and a meta-analysis of clinical trials. *Clin. Nutr.* 2019;38(3):1076–1091. doi:10.1016/j.clnu.2018.05.001

23 Trexler ET, Smith-Ryan AE, Stout JR, et al. International Society of Sports Nutrition Position Stand: beta-alanine. *J. Int. Soc. Sports Nutr.* 2015;12:30. Published 2015 Jul 15. doi:10.1186/s12970-015-0090-y

24 Artioli GG, Gualano B, Smith A, Stout J, Lancha AH Jr. Role of beta-alanine supplementation on muscle carnosine and exercise performance. *Med. Sci. Sports Exerc.* 2010;42(6):1162–1173. doi:10.1249/MSS.0b013e3181c74e38

25 Harris RC, Stellingwerff T. Effect of β-alanine supplementation on high-intensity exercise performance. *Nestle Nutr. Inst. Workshop Ser.* 2013;76:61–71. doi:10.1159/000350258

26 Chung W, Baguet A, Bex T, Bishop DJ, Derave W. Doubling of muscle carnosine concentration does not improve laboratory 1-hr cycling time-trial performance. *Int. J. Sport Nutr. Exerc. Metab.* 2014;24(3):315–324. doi:10.1123/ijsnem.2013-0125

27 Vitale K, Getzin A. Nutrition and supplement update for the endurance athlete: review and recommendations. *Nutrients* 2019;11(6):1289. Published 2019 Jun 7. doi:10.3390/nu11061289

28 Naderi A, Gobbi N, Ali A, et al. Carbohydrates and endurance exercise: a narrative review of a food first approach. *Nutrients* 2023;15(6):1367. Published 2023 Mar 11. doi:10.3390/nu15061367
29 Salvador AF, McKenna CF, Alamilla RA, et al. Potato ingestion is as effective as carbohydrate gels to support prolonged cycling performance. *J. Appl. Physiol. (1985)* 2019;127(6):1651–1659. doi:10.1152/japplphysiol.00567.2019
30 Williams MH. Vitamin supplementation and athletic performance. *Int. J. Vitam. Nutr. Res. Suppl.* 1989;30:163–191.
31 Yeung LK, Alschuler DM, Wall M, et al. Multivitamin supplementation improves memory in older adults: a randomized clinical trial. *Am. J. Clin. Nutr.* 2023;118(1):273–282. doi:10.1016/j.ajcnut.2023.05.011
32 van Dronkelaar C, van Velzen A, Abdelrazek M, et al. Minerals and sarcopenia; the role of calcium, iron, magnesium, phosphorus, potassium, selenium, sodium, and zinc on muscle mass, muscle strength, and physical performance in older adults: a systematic review. *J. Am. Med. Dir. Assoc.* 2018;19(1):6–11.e3. doi:10.1016/j.jamda.2017.05.026
33 van Dronkelaar C, Fultinga M, Hummel M, Kruizenga H, Weijs PJM, Tieland M. Minerals and sarcopenia in older adults: an updated systematic review. *J. Am. Med. Dir. Assoc.* 2023;24(8):1163–1172. doi:10.1016/j.jamda.2023.05.017
34 Hadžović-Džuvo A, Valjevac A, Lepara O, et al. Oxidative stress status in elite athletes engaged in different sport disciplines. *Bosn. J. Basic Med. Sci.* 2014;14(2):56–62. doi:10.17305/bjbms.2014.2262
35 Pingitore A, Lima GP, Mastorci F, et al. Exercise and oxidative stress: potential effects of antioxidant dietary strategies in sports. *Nutrition* 2015;31(7–8):916–922. doi:10.1016/j.nut.2015.02.005
36 Raghu G, Berk M, Campochiaro PA, et al. The multifaceted therapeutic role of *N*-acetylcysteine (NAC) in disorders characterized by oxidative stress. *Curr. Neuropharmacol.* 2021;19(8):1202–1224. doi:10.2174/1570159X19666201230144109
37 Šalamon Š, Kramar B, Marolt TP, Poljšak B, Milisav I. Medical and dietary uses of *N*-acetylcysteine. *Antioxidants (Basel)* 2019;8(5):111. Published 2019 Apr 28. doi:10.3390/antiox8050111
38 Fernández-Lázaro D, Domínguez-Ortega C, Busto N, et al. Influence of *N*-acetylcysteine supplementation on physical performance and laboratory biomarkers in adult males: a systematic review of controlled trials. *Nutrients* 2023;15(11):2463. Published 2023 May 25. doi:10.3390/nu15112463
39 Kumar P, Liu C, Suliburk J, et al. Supplementing glycine and *N*-acetylcysteine (GlyNAC) in older adults improves glutathione deficiency,

oxidative stress, mitochondrial dysfunction, inflammation, physical function, and aging hallmarks: a randomized clinical trial. *J. Gerontol. A Biol. Sci. Med. Sci.* 2023;78(1):75–89. doi:10.1093/gerona/glac135

40 Brownlee KK, Moore AW, Hackney AC. Relationship between circulating cortisol and testosterone: influence of physical exercise. *J. Sports Sci. Med.* 2005;4(1):76–83. Published 2005 Mar 1.

41 Khan SU, Jannat S, Shaukat H, et al. Stress induced cortisol release depresses the secretion of testosterone in patients with type 2 diabetes mellitus. *Clin. Med. Insights Endocrinol. Diabetes* 2023;16: 11795514221145841. Published 2023 Jan 3. doi:10.1177/1179551422114584

42 Baker WL, Karan S, Kenny AM. Effect of dehydroepiandrosterone on muscle strength and physical function in older adults: a systematic review. *J. Am. Geriatr. Soc.* 2011;59(6):997–1002. doi:10.1111/j.1532-5415.2011.03410.x

43 Kenny AM, Boxer RS, Kleppinger A, et al. Dehydroepiandrosterone combined with exercise improves muscle strength and physical function in frail older women. *J. Am. Geriatr. Soc.* 2010;58(9):1707–1714. doi:10.1111/j.1532-5415.2010.03019.x

44 Legrain S, Girard L. Pharmacology and therapeutic effects of dehydroepiandrosterone in older subjects. *Drugs Aging.* 2003;20(13):949–967. doi:10.2165/00002512-200320130-00001

45 Rutkowski K, Sowa P, Rutkowska-Talipska J, et al. Dehydroepiandrosterone (DHEA): hypes and hopes. *Drugs* 2014;74(11):1195–1207. doi:10.1007/s40265-014-0259-8

46 Collomp K, Buisson C, Gravisse N, et al. Effects of short-term DHEA intake on hormonal responses in young recreationally trained athletes: modulation by gender. *Endocrine* 2018;59(3):538–546. doi:10.1007/s12020-017-1514-z

47 Fernández-Lázaro D, Fernandez-Lazaro CI, Seco-Calvo J, et al. Effects of *Tribulus terrestris* L. on sport and health biomarkers in physically active adult males: a systematic review. *Int. J. Environ. Res. Public Health* 2022;19(15):9533. Published 2022 Aug 3. doi:10.3390/ijerph19159533

48 Fernández-Lázaro D, Mielgo-Ayuso J, Del Valle Soto M, Adams DP, González-Bernal JJ, Seco-Calvo J. The effects of 6 weeks of *Tribulus terrestris* L. supplementation on body composition, hormonal response, perceived exertion, and CrossFit® performance: a randomized, single-blind, placebo-controlled study. *Nutrients* 2021;13(11):3969. Published 2021 Nov 7. doi:10.3390/nu13113969

49 Kingsley M. Effects of phosphatidylserine supplementation on exercising humans. *Sports Med.* 2006;36(8):657–669. doi:10.2165/00007256-200636080-00003

50 Kingsley MI, Miller M, Kilduff LP, McEneny J, Benton D. Effects of phosphatidylserine on exercise capacity during cycling in active males. *Med. Sci. Sports Exerc.* 2006;38(1):64–71. doi:10.1249/01.mss.0000183195.10867.d0

51 Starks MA, Starks SL, Kingsley M, Purpura M, Jäger R. The effects of phosphatidylserine on endocrine response to moderate intensity exercise. *J. Int. Soc. Sports Nutr.* 2008;5:11. Published 2008 Jul 28. doi:10.1186/1550-2783-5-11

52 Heileson JL, Machek SB, Harris DR, et al. The effect of fish oil supplementation on resistance training-induced adaptations. *J. Int. Soc. Sports Nutr.* 2023;20(1):2174704. doi:10.1080/15502783.2023.2174704

53 Tsuchiya Y, Yanagimoto K, Nakazato K, Hayamizu K, Ochi E. Eicosapentaenoic and docosahexaenoic acids-rich fish oil supplementation attenuates strength loss and limited joint range of motion after eccentric contractions: a randomized, double-blind, placebo-controlled, parallel-group trial [published correction appears in Eur J Appl Physiol. 2016 Sep;116(9):1855-6]. *Eur. J. Appl. Physiol.* 2016;116(6):1179–1188. doi:10.1007/s00421-016-3373-3

54 Murphy CH, McGlory C. Fish oil for healthy aging: potential application to master athletes. *Sports Med.* 2021;51(Suppl 1):31–41. doi:10.1007/s40279-021-01509-7

55 Philpott JD, Witard OC, Galloway SDR. Applications of omega-3 polyunsaturated fatty acid supplementation for sport performance. *Res. Sports Med.* 2019;27(2):219–237. doi:10.1080/15438627.2018.1550401

56 Daily JW, Yang M, Park S. Efficacy of turmeric extracts and curcumin for alleviating the symptoms of joint arthritis: a systematic review and meta-analysis of randomized clinical trials. *J. Med. Food.* 2016;19(8):717–729. doi:10.1089/jmf.2016.3705

57 Zeng L, Yu G, Hao W, Yang K, Chen H. The efficacy and safety of *Curcuma longa* extract and curcumin supplements on osteoarthritis: a systematic review and meta-analysis. *Biosci. Rep.* 2021;41(6):BSR20210817. doi:10.1042/BSR20210817

58 Wu J, Lv M, Zhou Y. Efficacy and side effect of curcumin for the treatment of osteoarthritis: a meta-analysis of randomized controlled trials. *Pak. J. Pharm. Sci.* 2019;32(1):43–51.

59 Steven A Basham Ms, Waldman HS, Krings BM, et al. Effect of curcumin supplementation on exercise-induced oxidative stress, inflammation, muscle damage, and muscle soreness. *J. Diet Suppl.* 2020;17(4):401–414. doi:10.1080/19390211.2019.1604604

60 Serrata B. *LiverTox: Clinical and Research Information on Drug-Induced Liver Injury.* [Updated 2020 Nov 4]. Bethesda (MD): National Institute of

Diabetes and Digestive and Kidney Diseases, 2012. Available from: https://www.ncbi.nlm.nih.gov/books/NBK563692/

61 Siddiqui MZ. Boswellia serrata, a potential antiinflammatory agent: an overview. *Indian J. Pharm. Sci.* 2011;73(3):255–261. doi:10.4103/0250-474X.93507

62 Vitale KC, Hueglin S, Broad E. Tart cherry juice in athletes: a literature review and commentary. *Curr. Sports Med. Rep.* 2017;16(4):230–239. doi:10.1249/JSR.0000000000000385

63 Gao R, Chilibeck PD. Effect of tart cherry concentrate on endurance exercise performance: a meta-analysis. *J. Am. Coll. Nutr.* 2020;39(7):657–664. doi:10.1080/07315724.2020.1713246

64 Kuehl KS, Perrier ET, Elliot DL, Chesnutt JC. Efficacy of tart cherry juice in reducing muscle pain during running: a randomized controlled trial. *J. Int. Soc. Sports Nutr.* 2010;7:17. Published 2010 May 7. doi:10.1186/1550-2783-7-17

65 Kurtz JA, Vandusseldorp TA, Uken B, Otis J. Quercetin in sports and exercise: a review. *Int. J. Exerc. Sci.* 2023;16(2):1334–1384. Published 2023 Oct 1.

66 Kressler J, Millard-Stafford M, Warren GL. Quercetin and endurance exercise capacity: a systematic review and meta-analysis [published correction appears in Med Sci Sports Exerc. 2012 Mar;44(3):558-9]. *Med. Sci. Sports Exerc.* 2011;43(12):2396–2404. doi:10.1249/MSS.0b013e31822495a7

67 Pakulak A, Candow DG, Totosy de Zepetnek J, Forbes SC, Basta D. Effects of creatine and caffeine supplementation during resistance training on body composition, strength, endurance, rating of perceived exertion and fatigue in trained young adults. *J. Diet Suppl.* 2022;19(5):587–602. doi:10.1080/19390211.2021.1904085

68 Candow DG, Prokopidis K, Forbes SC, et al. Resistance exercise and creatine supplementation on fat mass in adults < 50 years of age: a systematic review and meta-analysis. *Nutrients* 2023;15(20):4343. Published 2023 Oct 12. doi:10.3390/nu15204343

69 Devries MC, Phillips SM. Creatine supplementation during resistance training in older adults-a meta-analysis. *Med. Sci. Sports Exerc.* 2014;46(6):1194–1203. doi:10.1249/MSS.0000000000000220

70 Grgic J, Pedisic Z, Saunders B, et al. International Society of Sports Nutrition position Stand: sodium bicarbonate and exercise performance. *J. Int. Soc. Sports Nutr.* 2021;18(1):61. Published 2021 Sep 9. doi:10.1186/s12970-021-00458-w

71 Peart DJ, Siegler JC, Vince RV. Practical recommendations for coaches and athletes: a meta-analysis of sodium bicarbonate use for athletic performance. *J. Strength Cond. Res.* 2012;26(7):1975–1983. doi:10.1519/JSC.0b013e3182576f3d

72 McNaughton LR, Gough L, Deb S, Bentley D, Sparks SA. Recent developments in the use of sodium bicarbonate as an ergogenic aid. *Curr. Sports Med. Rep.* 2016;15(4):233–244. doi:10.1249/JSR.0000000000000283

73 Guest NS, VanDusseldorp TA, Nelson MT, et al. International Society of Sports Nutrition Position Stand: caffeine and exercise performance. *J. Int. Soc. Sports Nutr.* 2021;18(1):1. Published 2021 Jan 2. doi:10.1186/s12970-020-00383-4

74 Pickering C, Grgic J. Caffeine and exercise: what next?. *Sports Med.* 2019;49(7):1007–1030. doi:10.1007/s40279-019-01101-0

75 Fiani B, Zhu L, Musch BL, et al. The neurophysiology of caffeine as a central nervous system stimulant and the resultant effects on cognitive function. *Cureus* 2021;13(5):e15032. Published 2021 May 14. doi:10.7759/cureus.15032

76 Martins GL, Guilherme JPLF, Ferreira LHB, et al. Caffeine and exercise performance: possible directions for definitive findings. *Front. Sports Act. Liv.* 2020;2:574854. doi:10.3389/fspor.2020.574854

77 Guest NS, VanDusseldorp TA, Nelson MT et al. International Society of Sports Nutrition Position Stand: caffeine and exercise performance. *J. Int. Soc. Sports Nutr.* 2021;18:1. doi:10.1186/s12970-020-00383-4

78 Tabrizi R, Saneei P, Lankarani KB, et al. The effects of caffeine intake on weight loss: a systematic review and dose-response meta-analysis of randomized controlled trials. *Crit. Rev. Food Sci. Nutr.* 2019;59(16):2688–2696. doi:10.1080/10408398.2018.1507996

79 Gonzalez AM, Townsend JR, Pinzone AG, Hoffman JR. Supplementation with nitric oxide precursors for strength performance: a review of the current literature. *Nutrients* 2023;15(3):660. Published 2023 Jan 28. doi:10.3390/nu15030660

80 Shannon OM, Clifford T, Seals DR, Craighead DH, Rossman MJ. Nitric oxide, aging and aerobic exercise: sedentary individuals to Master's athletes. *Nitric Oxide.* 2022;125–126:31–39. doi:10.1016/j.niox.2022.06.002

81 Vincent JB, Lukaski HC. Chromium. *Adv. Nutr.* 2018;9(4):505–506. doi:10.1093/advances/nmx021

82 Williams MH. Dietary supplements and sports performance: minerals. *J. Int. Soc. Sports Nutr.* 2005;2(1):43–49. Published 2005 Jun 11. doi:10.1186/1550-2783-2-1-43

83 Lefavi RG, Anderson RA, Keith RE, et al. Efficacy of chromium supplementation in athletes: emphasis on anabolism. *Int. J. Sport Nutr.* 1992;2(2):111–122. doi:10.1123/ijsn.2.2.111

84 Vincent JB. The potential value and toxicity of chromium picolinate as a nutritional supplement, weight loss agent and muscle development agent. *Sports Med.* 2003;33(3):213–230. doi:10.2165/00007256-200333030-00004

85 Huang H, Liao D, Zou Y, Chi H. The effects of chitosan supplementation on body weight and body composition: a systematic review and meta-analysis of randomized controlled trials. *Crit. Rev Food Sci. Nutr.* 2020;60(11):1815–1825. doi:10.1080/10408398.2019.1602822

86 Ylitalo R, Lehtinen S, Wuolijoki E, Ylitalo P, Lehtimäki T. Cholesterol-lowering properties and safety of chitosan. *Arzneimittelforschung.* 2002;52(1):1–7. doi:10.1055/s-0031-1299848

87 Guo W, Yi L, Zhou B, Li M. Chitosan modifies glycemic levels in people with metabolic syndrome and related disorders: meta-analysis with trial sequential analysis. *Nutr. J.* 2020;19(1):130. Published 2020 Dec 1. doi:10.1186/s12937-020-00647-4

88 Avois L, Robinson N, Saudan C, et al. Central nervous system stimulants and sport practice. *Br. J. Sports Med.* 2006;40 (Suppl 1):i16–i20. doi:10.1136/bjsm.2006.027557

89 Yoo HJ, Yoon HY, Yee J, Gwak HS. Effects of ephedrine-containing products on weight loss and lipid profiles: a systematic review and meta-analysis of randomized controlled trials. *Pharmaceuticals (Basel)* 2021;14(11):1198. Published 2021 Nov 22. doi:10.3390/ph14111198

90 World Anti-Doping Agency. The 2022 Prohibited List. 2021. https://www.wada-ama.org/sites/default/files/resources/files/2022list_final_en.pdf

91 Harty PS, Zabriskie HA, Erickson JL, et al. Multi-ingredient pre-workout supplements, safety implications, and performance outcomes: a brief review. *J. Int. Soc. Sports Nutr.* 2018;15(1):41. Published 2018 Aug 8. doi:10.1186/s12970-018-0247-6

92 Stratton MT, Siedler MR, Harty PS, et al. The influence of caffeinated and non-caffeinated multi-ingredient pre-workout supplements on resistance exercise performance and subjective outcomes. *J. Int. Soc. Sports Nutr.* 2022;19(1):126–149. Published 2022 Apr 4. doi:10.1080/15502783.2022.2060048

93 Strasser B, Wolters M, Weyh C, Krüger K, Ticinesi A. The effects of lifestyle and diet on gut microbiota composition, inflammation and muscle performance in our aging society. *Nutrients* 2021;13(6):2045. Published 2021 Jun 15. doi:10.3390/nu13062045

94 Mohr AE, Jäger R, Carpenter KC, et al. The athletic gut microbiota. *J. Int. Soc. Sports Nutr.* 2020;17(1):24. Published 2020 May 12. doi:10.1186/s12970-020-00353-w

95 Giron M, Thomas M, Dardevet D, Chassard C, Savary-Auzeloux I. Gut microbes and muscle function: can probiotics make our muscles stronger?. *J. Cachexia Sarcopenia Muscle* 2022;13(3):1460–1476. doi:10.1002/jcsm.12964

96 Jäger R, Mohr AE, Carpenter KC, et al. International Society of Sports Nutrition Position Stand: probiotics. *J. Int. Soc. Sports Nutr.* 2019;16(1):62. Published 2019 Dec 21. doi:10.1186/s12970-019-0329-0

97 Mohr AE, Jäger R, Carpenter KC, et al. The athletic gut microbiota. *J. Int. Soc. Sports Nutr.* 2020;17(1):24. Published 2020 May 12. doi:10.1186/s12970-020-00353-w

98 Di Dio M, Calella P, Pelullo CP, et al. Effects of probiotic supplementation on sports performance and performance-related features in athletes: a systematic review. *Int. J. Environ. Res. Public Health* 2023;20(3):2226. Published 2023 Jan 26. doi:10.3390/ijerph20032226

99 Bruyère O, Altman RD, Reginster JY. Efficacy and safety of glucosamine sulfate in the management of osteoarthritis: evidence from real-life setting trials and surveys. *Semin. Arthritis Rheum.* 2016;45(4 Suppl):S12–S17. doi:10.1016/j.semarthrit.2015.11.011

100 Messina OD, Vidal Wilman M, Vidal Neira LF. Nutrition, osteoarthritis and cartilage metabolism. *Aging Clin. Exp. Res.* 2019;31(6):807–813. doi:10.1007/s40520-019-01191-w

101 Nagaoka I, Tsuruta A, Yoshimura M. Chondroprotective action of glucosamine, a chitosan monomer, on the joint health of athletes. *Int. J. Biol. Macromol.* 2019;132:795–800. doi:10.1016/j.ijbiomac.2019.03.234

102 Meng Z, Liu J, Zhou N. Efficacy and safety of the combination of glucosamine and chondroitin for knee osteoarthritis: a systematic review and meta-analysis. *Arch. Orthop. Trauma Surg.* 2023;143(1):409–421. doi:10.1007/s00402-021-04326-9

103 Singh JA, Noorbaloochi S, MacDonald R, Maxwell LJ. Chondroitin for osteoarthritis. *Cochrane Database Syst. Rev.* 2015;1(1):CD005614. Published 2015 Jan 28. doi:10.1002/14651858.CD005614.pub2

104 Butawan M, Benjamin RL, Bloomer RJ. Methylsulfonylmethane: applications and safety of a novel dietary supplement. *Nutrients* 2017;9(3):290. Published 2017 Mar 16. doi:10.3390/nu9030290

105 van der Merwe M, Bloomer RJ. The influence of methylsulfonylmethane on inflammation-associated cytokine release before and following strenuous exercise. *J. Sports Med. (Hindawi Publ Corp).* 2016;2016:7498359. doi:10.1155/2016/7498359

106 Jagim AR, Harty PS, Erickson JL, et al. Prevalence of adulteration in dietary supplements and recommendations for safe supplement practices in sport. *Front. Sports Act. Living* 2023;5:1239121. Published 2023 Sep 29. doi:10.3389/fspor.2023.1239121

107 Lauritzen F. Dietary supplements as a major cause of anti-doping rule violations. *Front. Sports Act. Living* 2022;4:868228. Published 2022 Mar 25. doi:10.3389/fspor.2022.868228

108 Rocha T, Amaral JS, Oliveira MBPP. Adulteration of dietary supplements by the illegal addition of synthetic drugs: a review. *Compr. Rev. Food Sci. Food Saf.* 2016;15(1):43–62. doi:10.1111/1541-4337.12173

11

Putting It All Together

11.1 Introduction

Now that we have covered the basic theories behind the creation of a nutritional plan let us turn out attention to putting this information into clinical action. In this chapter, we will discuss how to work up an athlete's case from initial contact through to the development of a nutritional strategy. In our scenario, we will be discussing the case of Steve, a 50-year-old male powerlifter. Although this case is based on a specific athlete and their presentation, the information in this chapter could be used for any athlete to be able to tailor their nutritional plan for their needs.

11.2 Nutritional Assessment

Nutritional assessment begins before the first visit, ideally, at the point that the visit is scheduled. Steve was asked to fill out a food diary in which he records the foods eaten, the amounts of food eaten, cooking methods, body weight, sleep, hydration, and exercises performed. He was also asked to fill out a food frequency questionnaire to get an idea of dietary patterns overall. As previously discussed, this information gives an idea of the foods that were consumed as well as any trends in his history. At the initial visit, Steve's assessment included a history, basic anthropometric measurements, and bodyfat measurements using a bioelectric impedance machine. More advanced nutritional assessments like sweat testing and indirect calorimetry were not selected to be performed at this time but will be considered for future evaluation if progress is not being made toward the athlete's goals. The results of this assessment, including a brief synopsis of the food diary, and the food frequency questionnaire can be found in the following text.

Sports Nutrition for Masters Athletes, First Edition. Peter G. Nickless.
© 2025 John Wiley & Sons, Inc. Published 2025 by John Wiley & Sons, Inc.

11.2.1 Case Example

11.2.1.1 Significant History
Steve reports that he has been powerlifting for 20 years. His progress has stalled lately, reporting that he struggles to lift the same weights at competitions with no increases in his one rep max for the past two years. Steve reports a chronic history of mild episodic low back pain, for which he sees a Chiropractor twice a month and mild joint pain in both of his knees. Steve has no other reported health conditions and no limitations in his ability to perform exercise. Steve has no relevant family history of major diseases. Steve does not drink fluids during his workouts.

11.2.1.2 Basic Anthropometric Measurements
Steve-
Age: 50 years old
Sex: Male
Height: 74 in.
Weight: 100 kg
Waist: 36 in.
Neck circumference: 14 in.
Bodyfat (US Navy measurement method): 21%
Bodyfat (hydrostatic weighing): 15%

11.2.1.3 Food Diary and FFQ Analysis
Steve typically consumes convenience foods as snacks daily, including potato chips and commercially available protein bars. Steve typically has eggs, toast, and coffee for breakfast and some type of sandwich (the type varies) for lunch with chips and a cookie. During the midday, Steve typically has a protein shake (1 scoop 19 g whey concentrate) mixed with water. For dinner, Steve often has steak, a vegetable, and a potato. Two times weekly he will eat pasta with either meatballs or a meat sauce. Steve has ice cream three to four days per week as dessert. Steve drinks diet cola three to five servings per day and coffee three servings per day. Steve drinks very little water. FFQ supports that these foods are representative of Steves's typical diet.

11.2.1.4 Macronutrient Averages
Calories 2400
Carbohydrates 360 g (60%)
Protein 120 g (20%)
Fat 53 g (20%)
Fiber 12 g

11.2.1.5 Current Supplements
Protein powder 19 g/serving 90 calories
Multivitamin/multimineral 1 per day
Creatine monohydrate 5 g/day

11.2.1.6 Exercise Information
Steve typically works out three days per week. Workouts consist of strength training at intensities ranging from 70% to 90% with higher intensities up to 95% of his one rep max performed monthly. Steve only performs a one rep max at competitions. Workouts typically last one and a half hour, consisting of sets of three to five repetitions with a minimum of three minutes in between sets. Steve does a 5-minute warmup on the elliptical machine and stretches for 10 minutes after lifting weights.

11.2.1.7 Initial Analysis
Steve has an intense workout schedule with a focus on anaerobic activities. Despite the fact that he works out for over an hour and a half, there is ample rest to recover. His workouts largely focus heavily on the phosphagen and on anaerobic glycolytic pathways. He currently consumes 2400 calories which is too low for his current presentation, as well as too little protein and carbohydrates. He consumes too many convenience foods, which may have some negative impact on inflammation, particular the foods containing refined carbohydrates and sugars. He does not eat enough fiber which could impact his general health and his microbiome. His current lack of progress in powerlifting makes sense, given his initial presentation. He likely lacks the nutrients needed to perform and recover. This is supported by his self-report that he struggles to lift the same weights with no increases in his maximal lifts in two years.

11.3 Establishing Dietary Goals

Initiating a performance dietary plan with an athlete must begin with at least some thought about the athlete's goals. While all athletes, and all people for that matter, could benefit from an individually designed nutritional plan based on their individual needs, athletes should know why they are starting a nutritional plan at the outset. This will help them to maintain focus and follow the plan as written. The best way to do this is to have the athlete establish goals. Ask the athlete to write out what it is that they want to accomplish as they embark on this journey. Are they trying to become leaner while maintaining muscle mass so they can improve their running times? Are they trying to go up a weight class in a strength sport so that they can improve their competitive lifts? These are important decisions as they will shape the rest of what you do when collaborating with them. Having the athlete write out their goals is important for two reasons. First, these goals are something that should guide the overarching framework of the nutritional strategy and, accordingly, should be referred to regularly. For the nutritional practitioner, these will be used to guide your strategy and be used as a patient education tool so that you can tie your plan to the expected result. For the athlete, this is an effective way to solidify what they are trying to achieve and something they can refer to as they progress to see how they are achieving their goals. The second reason you should have the athlete write down their goals is that you, as the nutritional professional, can help focus the athlete on something achievable. Lofty goals are great but sometimes need to be focused on more manageable parts. These parts can ultimately lead to the lofty goal eventually. Writing goals down helps the nutritional practitioner to be able to assess and focus their plan on them. This may mean having a difficult conversation with the athlete if their goals are unrealistic or even unhealthy. On the other hand, if the athlete's goal is achievable but complex, for example, gaining a substantial amount of muscle while losing body fat, you may be able to break this goal into sub-goals that can be more easily achieved, such as an initial phase of a muscle building followed by a fat loss phase. The overall outcome is still achieving the overall goal, but you have provided some direction and clarification on how to accomplish this. As you progress with the nutritional plan, you will want to return to these goals to help focus the athlete and progressively refine them more. If, for example, the athlete wants to improve their body composition, you may go back to this every month to see how their body composition changes, but since your result is not going to be a permanent diet to lower body fat. The refinement could include a target body fat percentage and a plan to start thinking of establishing the next goal, such as maintaining this body composition for a period.

11.3.1 Case Example

Let us look at our example: Steve is a 50-year-old male athlete with 15% body fat and weighs 100 kg at 74 in. He currently competes in powerlifting and wants to move from the 220 lb. to the 242 lb. weight class. His goal is to maintain his current body fat percentage but he wants to be at the top of the class and weigh a full 242 lbs. He plans to compete at a master's level national competition in nine months but may do some local competitions in the meantime. As we examine his goals, we can see that we need a diet to increase both body weight and lean body mass, as just gaining weight may not maintain the desired body fat percentage. There are several ways to achieve this goal, but I suggest using a three-phase strategy. The first phase would be to increase overall mass with a focus on building muscle but without focusing too much on body fat percentage. The second phase would involve reducing body fat while maintaining as much of the newly acquired muscle as possible. The third phase would be for the athlete to maintain this new body composition while putting the finishing touches on his training for the competition. Additionally, this is a suitable time to discuss the goal in terms of how realistic it is. While the athlete should be able to increase his muscle mass while maintaining 15% body fat over a large period of time, particularly if breaking it down into manageable subgoals, it is unrealistic that he will be a full 242 lb. athlete with 15% body fat on the day of competition in only nine months. At his current weight and body fat percentage, his lean body mass is 187 lbs. at 15% body fat and 242 lbs. he would need to increase his lean body mass to 206 lbs. It is unrealistic for a drug-free older adult male to expect to put on 19 lbs. of lean mass quickly. We can get him to gain the weight, but he may put on more fat than he would want. So, a modification of the goal should be to be in the weight class (between 221 and 242 lbs.) at 15% body fat but not at that exact weight of 242 lbs.

11.4 Establishing Performance Metrics

Now that we have established goals for the nutritional strategy, it is important that the athlete and nutritional provider work together to establish the metrics that will be used to define the successes or failures of the nutritional strategy. These metrics are the measurements that we use to evaluate progress toward the goal and can be used to inform if there is a need to alter the nutritional strategy. Think of them as checkpoints on the way to reaching your goal. The metrics can be highly individual and can take the form of physical performance metrics, such as 40-yard sprint time, objective physical metrics, such as body fat percentage, or subjective assessments, such as the athlete's perception of energy or performance. I do not advocate subjective assessments alone as they can change daily based on a variety of factors. Still, I do recommend that subjective performance goals be evaluated along with something objective to get a more complete picture. The more of these metrics used then the more complete a picture we can see of how the athlete is progressing. Let us, for example, take a metric like the 5 km run time. If the athlete's 5 km run time remains the same or sees only a minimal improvement after four to six weeks following the nutritional plan, we could interpret this as a diet failure. Now, if we add in the subjective assessment that the athlete felt the run took less of a toll on him or her and the athlete had less soreness following the exertion, we start to see that there may have been some benefit to the strategy, which may be worth continuing. Adding an additional metric like body weight may provide even more information. In the aforementioned example, if the athlete's 5 km time did not change but felt they recovered more quickly and lost 4 lbs. of body weight over four weeks, we can clearly see that the diet has had a benefit. We can now make better plans moving forward with this information to refine the strategy based on how effective it has or has not been.

11.4.1 Case Example

In looking at our example of the 50-year-old powerlifter, we can see some obvious physical metrics to use, such as body weight since the athlete wants to increase his weight; body fat percentage is another metric since the athlete wants to maintain 15% body fat. We then also have performance metrics based on the athlete's sport. The squat, bench press, and deadlift are the contested events used in the sport and can act as a good metric to determine success. The athlete would likely not be lifting to their maximum many times during their training. Still, there will likely be times when their training routine will call for either a repetition or poundage test, and this information can prove valuable. If these tests indicate either increases in weight lifted or number of repetitions performed, then there is an indication of performance improvement. In the realm of subjective assessments, we can consider the athlete's perception of effort as a measurement of success. A weight lifted with difficulty in the past feeling lighter is a good example; the athlete's perception of their recovery, their energy levels, and their sleep will also be useful information to help provide information to evaluate if the nutritional strategy has seen some success. In Steve's case, we will use the objective metrics of success: body weight, body fat, weight lifted, and repetitions lifted. We will also use the subjective metric of perceived exertion during heavy lifting. Steve will record these daily in his food diary to be examined during reevaluations.

11.5 Creating the Nutritional Plan

Now that we have established a goal for the nutritional strategy and determined the metrics by which we will evaluate whether it has been successful, we can start writing the nutritional plan to help the athlete achieve their goals. The creation of a nutritional strategy will start with the determination of the caloric needs of the athlete.

11.6 Determining Caloric Needs

After we have solidified the goals of the athlete and the metrics that will be used to evaluate if we are moving toward achieving these goals, it is time to start creating the nutritional plan. This begins with determining the caloric requirements needed to support the athlete's goals. These caloric requirements need to consider both the physiological needs for survival and the activities asked of the athlete. Adequate calories are essential to ensure athletes can perform and recover from their athletic training. A calorie is defined as the amount of energy required to raise one gram of water one degree Celsius. In more real-world terms, calories are a unit of energy that can act like a form of currency. This currency can be used to fuel the energy systems needed for survival and performance. If the athlete were to eat too few calories, they would have a negative energy balance, which can result in weight loss, decreased recovery, decreased immunity, and reduced performance. Consuming too many calories would result in a positive energy balance, resulting in unwanted weight gain, which can impact performance negatively and potentially impact chronic disease processes. Regardless of age, the key for any athlete is to find the minimal caloric level that will allow for optimal recovery and performance with no excess. As athletes age, their metabolisms change, often slowing down, which requires a more frequent assessment of caloric needs. This chapter will examine the factors that will determine the appropriate caloric requirements.

11.6.1 Total Caloric Requirements

The determination of caloric requirements can be boiled down to the following equation (Figure 11.1).

We will be exploring the elements that contribute to the total caloric requirement in the sections below.

11.6.2 Basal Metabolic Rate

The resting metabolic rate (RMR) or the basal metabolic rate (BMR) are the energy requirements (in calories) needed to maintain the

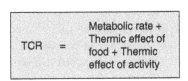

Figure 11.1 Total caloric requirement.

physiological processes needed for survival. This does not include any movement or activity but simply keeping the individual alive. The BMR is slightly different from the RMR as the BMR is assessed with the individual at waking in the morning after a fast, while the RMR, on the other hand, is assessed after a meal with no physical activity in the previous 12 hours. This difference in how the two are measured means that the RMR would be slightly higher and more accurately reflect an individual's caloric needs with at least some movement [1]. In this chapter, we will use the BMR in the determination of caloric needs for the athlete and then add the effect of activity to this calculation. The BMR accounts for approximately 60–75% of the daily caloric requirements.

The BMR is not the same for everyone and must be calculated individually for every athlete and take into consideration several factors. Body size, for example, is an important factor to consider in determining the BMR, as the larger the individual, the greater the caloric needs to maintain cellular processes. The greater the body weight, the larger the BMR. Body habitus is another important factor. Since body fat consumes fewer calories, the higher the lean body mass, the higher the BMR. This is largely due to the increased caloric demand required to maintain the extra muscle mass (note: not all BMR formulae take body composition into account). Height is another factor that will impact the BMR, as the larger the surface area of the individual, the greater the BMR. Looking at the height and weight of an individual can also act to consider the body composition of an individual. A 200 lb. individual who is 6'2" will typically be leaner than the same body weight for a 5'2" individual. Age is also important to consider, as the BMR will decline as a person ages. This is due to the physiologic changes that are due to aging that result in a decrease in the athlete's metabolic requirements. The loss of muscle mass that commonly occurs during aging is an example of a physiological change that would decrease the BMR. This is a particularly important consideration when working with older athletes. Gender is another important consideration, as factors like endocrine differences, body composition differences, and bone density differences will all have an impact on the BMR. Other factors will impact the BMR, such as certain physiological considerations such as endocrine disorders or some chronic diseases. Supplementation can also impact caloric needs. The effects of caffeine, for example, will increase the number of calories burned and accordingly raise the caloric requirements to maintain body weight slightly.

Many methods can be employed in determining the BMR, ranging from mathematical calculations to more accurate metabolic testing such as indirect calorimetry. The determination of the BMR is only the first step in the determination of the caloric requirements of an athlete. The next step would be to determine the impact that activity and eating have on the caloric requirements of the athlete. We do this by examining the thermic effect of activity (TEA) and the thermic effect of food (TEF).

11.6.3 The Thermic Effect of Activity

The TEA is the effect of athletic and nonathletic activity on caloric requirements. These energy requirements often contribute less to the total energy needs than BMR. The TEA becomes a factor as the individual moves from the resting state. The more active the individual, the higher the contribution of TEA to caloric requirements. This activity can come in several forms, such as activities of daily living, occupational duties, or athletic training and competition. A variety of factors will impact the effect of specific activities on the total requirement. For example, the intensity of the exercise, duration of exercise, and size of the person performing the exercise are important considerations when looking at the TEA. For this reason, the TEA is based on the caloric effect per hour per kg of body weight. Jogging, for example, is 7 kcal/h/kg, so a 100 kg individual (220 lbs.) would burn 700 calories/h while a 75 kg (165 lbs.) individual would burn 525 calories in the same time frame. Running at a pace of 10 mph will burn 16 kcal/h/kg, so the same 100 kg individual will burn 1600 kcal, and the 75 kg individual will burn 1200 kcal. The percentage contribution that the TEA will have on the total daily energy requirements largely depends on the individual's activity level and will account for a larger percentage of the energy requirements of an athlete when compared to a nonathlete. Performance declines seen with age may be essential for determining the TEA, as the exercise factors used must be adjusted to account for performance.

11.6.4 The Thermic Effect of Food

The TEF refers to the impact of diet on an individual's energy requirements. Simply put, the TEF refers to the impact of eating on energy needs. This is due to the increased energy demands to process different types of food. Generally speaking, the harder the body must work to digest and assimilate a meal, the larger the TEF. The TEF of food typically contributes approximately 10% to the total caloric requirements. This would mean that someone with a caloric requirement of 2000 calories will burn 200 calories by simply eating. Indicating that the larger the caloric consumption, the more calories burned. Keep in mind that the effect is a small percentage of energy requirements, so overeating will increase these requirements, but it is not a suitable weight loss strategy. The actual macronutrient makeup of the food can have an impact on the TEF. Protein, for example, takes up the largest amount of energy to metabolize, followed by carbohydrates and then fat. A diet that is higher in protein would, therefore, have a higher TEF when compared to a higher-fat diet. This does not consider the macronutrient needs of different athletes for optimal performance but simply the impact of these nutrients on the total energy expenditure. Athletes focused on body composition may use the TEF to their advantage in designing their diet plan. Still, most athletes will want to design their diet plan based on optimal performance rather than maximizing the TEF. Bodybuilding being one possible exception to this general rule.

11.6.5 Determining the Basal Metabolic Rate

There are a variety of equations that can be used to determine the BMR for athletes. Among these, the most reliable are the Harris–Benedict equation, the Mifflin–St. Jeor equation, and the Katch–Mcardle equation [2, 3]. See Figure 11.2.

Some of the common characteristics of the different equations for caloric requirements are that they all consider both the height and weight of the athlete in question. The Harris–Benedict equation and the Mifflin–St. Jeor equations will also consider the athlete's age, whereas an equation like Katch–Mcardle will not. The Katch–Mcardle equation also does not differentiate gender. These are essential considerations because when looking at both the Harris–Benedict equation and Mifflin–St. Jeor that the impact of age is a reduction in the BMR. What this means, in effect, is that as we age, our BMR will reduce when using these equations. The amount of this reduction differs depending on the equation used, but both equations consider this factor. So, while discussing all three equations mentioned, it is crucial to consider that only the equations that consider age truly apply to

---

Harris–Benedict Equation

Male BMR: = 66.4730 + (13.7516 × weight in kg) + (5.0033 × height in cm) − (6.7550 × age in years)
Female BMR: = 655.0955 + (9.5634 × weight in kg) + (1.8496 × height in cm) − (4.6756 × age in years)

Mifflin–St. Jeor

Male BMR: (10 × weight in kg) + (6.25 × height in cm) − (5 × age in years) + 5
Female BMR: (10 × weight in kg) + (6.25 × height in cm) − (5 × age in years) − 161

Katch–Mcardle

BMR = 370 + (21.6 × lean body mass (kg))

Figure 11.2 BMR formulae. *Source:* Joseph et al. [2] and Jagim et al. [3].

an aging athletic population. Part of the reasoning for the reduction based on age in BMR is that as we age, our muscle mass declines, which will impact our BMR. The Katch–Mcardle equation is based on the body composition more than the athlete's age, height, and total weight. In this regard, they are attempting to consider the age-related loss of lean body mass indirectly. Equally, since the other equations are based on height, weight, and age, they indirectly attempt to account for body composition. There are benefits and drawbacks to all three equations mentioned, and when working with athletes, you may find that you have a preference and will work with one equation over another. These equations represent a starting point in estimating the BMR and are suitable in the absence of more advanced testing [2, 3].

11.6.6 Activity Multiplier

The calculation of both the TEA and the TEF is the most accurate method of determining the non-BMR contributions to the total energy requirements of the athlete. This calculation may be difficult and time-consuming when working with athletes, particularly as factors such as the TEA and TEF may change frequently. Another method to determine the non-BMR contributions to caloric need is to generalize using an estimation. To accomplish this, we can use something called an activity multiplier. This is a number based on the individual's activity levels on the aggregate. So, while the training load may fluctuate weekly or even daily, this estimate can be used as an average of these factors. The activity multiplier is multiplied by the BMR to determine the overall caloric requirements. This activity multiplier is a constant that is then multiplied by the BMR to determine the caloric requirements of an individual. The more active the individual, the higher the activity multiplier. A sedentary individual, for example, will have an activity multiplier of 1.2, while a moderately active male will have an activity multiplier of 1.8. So, if we take two individuals, one sedentary and one moderately active, both with a BMR of 1200, we get total caloric requirements of 1440 and 2160, respectively. Interestingly, the activity multipliers do not change based on factors such as age or body composition, only based on activity and sex. Therefore, their application is an estimate at best and there will need to be adjustments to the caloric requirements based on how the athlete responds to the dietary plan [2–4] (Figure 11.3).

	Males	Females
Sedentary	1.2	1.2
Light	1.5	1.5
Moderate	1.8	1.7
Heavy	2.1	1.8

Figure 11.3 Activity multipliers.
Source: Data from Burke and Deakin [4].

11.6.7 Case Example

- Steve is a 50-year-old male 100 kg, 74 in. (187.96) weight workout three to four days per week 15% BF
  - **Harris Benedict Equation**
    - BMR = 66.4730 + (13.7516 × 100) + (5.0033 × 188) − (6.7550 × 50)
    - BMR = 2044.5 calories
  - **Mifflin–St. Jeor**
    - BMR = (10 × 100) + (6.25 × 188) − (5 × 50) + 5
    - BMR = 1930 calories
  - **Katch-Mcardle BMR Formula:**
    - BMR = 370 + (21.6 × 85)
    - BMR = 2206 calories

Average of all three equations 2060 calories

Since the athlete Steve is a light to moderately active powerlifter, training three to four days per week at one and a half hours with long rest periods, an activity multiplier of 1.6 would be a good starting point. Using the Harris–Benedict BMR value of 2044.5 calories and multiplying it by 1.6, we would get a total caloric requirement of 3271 calories per day to maintain his body weight. This is 871 more calories than Steve is currently eating.

Note: when using the activity multiplier, base it on the actual activity of the athlete, not their planned activity; for this, use the training journal if possible.

11.6.8 Alternate Methods for Calculation of Caloric Need

11.6.8.1 Cunningham Formula

The Cunningham formula is a simplified formula that can be used to determine caloric needs. This formula is based solely on the lean body mass (LBM). It is simply total caloric requirement (TCR) = 500 + (22 * LBM). In this case, an athlete with an LBM of 100 kg will have a TCR of 500 + (22 * 100) or 2700 calories. The use of lean body mass to determine the amount of calories an athlete needs carries a few flaws. Specifically, in that it does not take the gender or the age of the athlete into account. Additionally, since the LBM is used to calculate the equation, there is variation based on the total body fat. If we looked at two individuals with the same LBM and one had a 15% body fat and the other had 40%, the larger individual would expend more calories in just moving around throughout the day. So, there would be wide variations between the caloric determinations made by the Harris–Benedict formula, for example, compared to the Cunningham formula [3].

11.6.8.2 Rule of Thumb

Bodybuilding magazines of the 1980s popularized a few generalized rule-of-thumb methods. These rule-of-thumb methods have been passed down over the years, for example, the caloric requirement to lose body weight is 10 calories/lb. of body weight. This would mean a 200 lb. athlete could lose weight on a 2000-calorie diet. The caloric requirements to gain body weight are approximately 20 calories/lb., so a 200-lb male athlete will need 4000 calories to maintain body weight. The issue with generalizations like this is that they tend to coincide nicely with the formulas for athletes in the 20–30 age range who work with weights at a rate of three to four days per week. Unfortunately, they do not take differing athletic schedules and training routines and, most importantly, are not personalized to both age and sex. A rule of thumb like this is of little value to someone working with a master's athlete due to the lack of specificity. While I see some value in these alternative methods for a younger athletic population, specifically between the ages of 18 and 35, they are more just quick estimates of caloric requirement. They are not personalized and not applicable to master athletes. If a nutritional practitioner were to consider using this type of calculation method to determine caloric needs for an athlete of any age. In that case, care must be taken to evaluate the athlete's response to the dietary changes, and adjustments must be made to accommodate any undesired effects of the diet.

Regardless of the formula used, monitoring the athlete's response to the dietary plan related to their performance goals is important. If the athlete, for example, is looking to maintain their body weight while focusing on their performance. The athlete should be monitored not only for changes in performance as well as for changes in body weight. As these approaches are estimates only, they serve as an educated starting point for the determination of the caloric requirements of the athlete. As the athlete follows the diet, monitoring performance and/or weight will help identify any issues and needs for corrections. If, for example, an athlete's determined total caloric need is 2700 calories to maintain their weight while optimizing their performance and the athlete is slowly gaining weight by approximately a pound every three weeks, we can assume that the caloric determination was overestimated. This weight gain does not correlate to the athlete's stated goals and could result in a performance loss in a sport that relies on a high power-to-weight ratio. On the other hand, if this athlete were in a sport where gaining weight is not an issue, and their performance increased due to this gain, then this may be a good time to reassess goals with the athlete and consider allowing the short-term weight gain as long as performance improves.

11.6.9 Case Example

In the case of Steve, our 50-year-old athlete, we have an established goal of gaining weight, preferably muscle, to compete in a heavier weight class. We established that the goal for this athlete would be broken into three sub-goals, with the first being a bulking phase where the athlete will be trying to gain weight and muscle. During this phase, we want to increase the caloric requirements for the athlete to provide him with the nutritional material needed to gain weight. As we assess the metrics during this phase, we will determine if the athlete is gaining weight quickly enough or too quickly and accumulating too much body fat. At this time, the caloric requirements will be adapted based on the athlete's response, and as the athlete gains weight, there will be a need to reassess and add more calories. In the next sub-goal phase, we must reverse this and reduce calories to lose body fat.

In phase 1, Steve will add approximately 500 additional calories per day to increase his body weight. We are adding only an additional 500 calories to the above caloric requirement so that we can raise his weight slowly to avoid any unnecessary body fat accumulation. Steve will start with 3771 calories/day.

11.7 Determination of Macronutrient Needs

Now that we have figured out how many calories will be needed for this athlete, we need to take the time to determine the macronutrient breakdown that this athlete will need to fuel his training plan for the upcoming national powerlifting meet. The Acceptable Macronutrient Distribution range could be used but would hardly be specific to the individual athlete. Instead, we need to look at the nutritional recommendations of master's athletes for each of the macronutrients.

We will start off with protein, as it is the backbone for muscle building and essential for the recovery of this athlete from his training. Protein recommendations were covered in detail in Chapter 4, so I will not go into as much detail here but will use the ISSN protein recommendations of 1.4–1.6 g of protein per kg of body weight. In the case of this athlete, as an older athlete, I will start at the higher number as protein becomes more important for older athletes.

11.7.1 Case Example

Using Steve's current weight of 100 kg of body weight and multiplying this by 1.6 g/kg, we get 160 g of protein a day minimum to start. One hundred sixty grams of protein daily will equal 640 calories, at a rate of 4 calories/g of protein. This, of course, should be made of high-quality protein as discussed previously.

Now that we have determined the protein needs of our case example, we should look at determining the carbohydrate needs this athlete will need to be able to achieve his goals. As we have said in Chapter 4, unless we specifically use a low carbohydrate strategy, carbohydrates are an important macronutrient for fueling the athlete and providing the energy needed for recovery from sport. The amount of carbohydrates will be different depending on the athletic event being trained for or contested.

11.7.2 Case Example

Using the ISSN guidelines, Steve the powerlifter, will need 5–7 g/kg of body weight. This number was selected as moderate intensity, which most closely fits the typical workout. In Steve's case, we will use 5 g/kg as our baseline carbohydrate. So, for this 100-kg athlete, you will have him consume 500 g of carbohydrates, which, at 4 calories per g, will be 2000 calories daily.

Taking the protein requirements of 640 calories (or 160 g) and the carbohydrate requirements of 2000 calories (or 500 g), you get 2640 of the 3271 calories of the total caloric requirements (determined earlier in the chapter). This leaves 631 calories remaining to satisfy the daily requirements. As there are no other macronutrients, all these calories are to be used to meet the daily fat requirements. If you divide the 631 calories by 9 calories per g of fat, you get 70 g of fat. This would have our basic macronutrient breakdown as 640 calories (160 g) from protein, 2000 calories (500 g) from carbohydrates, and 631 calories (70 g) from fat.

This is the macronutrient breakdown needed to maintain the current body weight of 100 kg and not an increase to 110 kg or 242 lbs. This would require that you increase the calories to gain the weight. There is some debate about how many calories should be added when trying to put on weight intentionally. Too many calories will cause a faster weight gain and add too much body fat. Too few calories, and you risk not achieving the goal. Every 500 calories added above the athlete's maintenance requirement should equal approximately 1 lb. of body weight gained. This is a general estimate as weight gain is nonlinear and can rarely be predicted accurately. I recommend Steve not exceed this caloric increase to start to limit the amount of unneeded fat gain. It is expected that Steve will gain some fat during the plan's first phase, but this should ideally be kept to a minimum. This 500-calorie increase would bring our caloric allotment up to 3771 calories daily. As for the macronutrient breakdown, I suggest a ratio of approximately 50% carbohydrate, 35% fat, and 15% protein for these additional calories. In this case, we would have an additional 250 calories or 63 g of carbohydrates, 175 calories or 19 g of fat, and 75 calories or 19 g of protein. This brings the macronutrient totals to 563 g carbohydrates, 179 g protein, and 89 g fat. The athlete should start with this macronutrient distribution, and their progress should be monitored to ensure that they are both gaining weight, not too much fat and that they are performing well in their training program. In addition to this Steve will be recommended to increase his fiber intake to 38 g/day.

11.8 Determination of Micronutrient Needs

The determination of micronutrient needs is a little less straightforward compared to the formulas for macronutrient determination. In general, we need to take the above macronutrient strategy and suggest foods that provide all the micronutrient requirements that a master athlete would need to compete in a specific sport. Ideally, we should look at the micronutrients being consumed in the diet currently and examine any lab work that may show what nutrients the athlete may be deficient in. Additionally, any presenting concerns found during the history could give an indication as to the potential deficiencies in micronutrients the athlete may be experiencing. In the absence of lab work we should make sure the diet recommended is complete in the foods that will provide enough of the micronutrients needed and have a greater focus on micronutrients that would be specifically limited in this athlete based on presentation and sport.

11.8.1 Case Example

In this case, we have a food frequency questionnaire that does show limited fruit and vegetable consumption, but Steve is taking a daily multivitamin so he is likely not going to be deficient in many micronutrients. On the other hand, as a 50-year-old powerlifter, there is a concern that Steve needs to get enough calcium, magnesium, vitamin D, iron, vitamin B12, potassium, and antioxidants (vitamin A, E, zinc, selenium, etc.). See Chapter 5 on micronutrients for information on food sources.

11.9 Developing a Hydration Strategy

Now that we have determined the caloric, macro-, and micronutrient needs to fuel the athlete for optimal performance, it is important to tailor a hydration plan to meet their individual needs based on their personal characteristics and athletic event competed in. The determination of a focus hydration plan for the athlete is important for optimal performance. A full description of the development of a hydration plan was discussed in Chapter 7, but simply put, we will use the following calculations three to four hours before the workout 5–7 ml/kg of water, during the workout 0.3–2.4 ml/kg per hour, and after the workout 1.25–1.5 ml/kg of water.

11.9.1 Case Example

In the case of Steve, the powerlifter, we see that his assessments show he does not drink enough fluids currently and would perform better if he were to get a more focused hydration plan. In this case, Steve would need the following.

A daily overall intake of approximately 3.7 l daily (peri-workout hydration is included in this amount)
500 ml two to four hours before the workout
100 ml/h during the workout (sipped over the time period)
125 ml within an hour of the workout.

11.10 Establishing a Peri-workout Nutrition Plan

In order to fuel the athlete for optimal performance, it is important to develop a peri-workout nutritional plan. This plan should be targeted to the anticipated needs of the athlete to perform and recover from their training or event. The macronutrients consumed as part of the peri-workout nutritional plan are part of the macronutrient plan and not in addition to it.

11.10.1 Case Example

In the case of Steve, the powerlifter, the following peri-workout suggestions should provide the fuel needed for performance and recovery:
Pre-workout nutrition
A meal consisting of
25 g protein
150 g complex carbohydrate source, for example, sweet potatoes
Pre-workout hydration from above
Intra-workout nutrition
60 g carbohydrate (higher glycemic source) as part of the intra-workout hydration plan

Post-workout nutrition
25 g protein
100 g carbohydrate (mixture of simple and complex sugars)
5 g creatine
Post-workout hydration plan from above

11.11 Establishing a Targeted Supplementation Plan

The selection of supplementation is the final component of the development of a sound nutritional plan. As mentioned in the Chapter 10 on supplementation, the selection of supplements needs to be focused on the goals of the athlete and how to best support the athlete for optimal performance.

11.11.1 Case Example

As a powerlifter Steve has several goals for supplementation, muscle building and recovery, micronutrient replenishment, hormonal support, and legal ergogenic aids. Additionally, because Steve has been dealing with knee pain, some supplements to help control inflammation and support joint health may be useful. To this end, Steve would benefit from a protein supplement, creatine monohydrate, phosphatidylserine, tribulus terrestris, fish oil, glucosamine, chondroitin, MSM, citrulline, nitric oxide, and a multivitamin just to name a few. Collectively, this would likely be too much for Steve to take at one time and this many supplements would be counterproductive. I will start with a basic supplement plan for Steve and build if the desired outcomes are not being achieved. In this case, I would recommend Steve start with the following and add supplements if needed:

Protein powder (whey isolate) 20 g 2×/day as part of the macronutrient needs
Fish oil 2 g/day as part of the macronutrient needs
Creatine monohydrate 10 g/day
Multivitamin/multimineral
Citrulline 5 g/day
Glucosamine sulfate 1500 mg and chondroitin sulfate 1200 mg

Steve will start at this overall strategy; he will be instructed to keep a food diary that records his food choices, amounts eaten, times, eaten, body weight, fluid intake, supplement intake, a record of physical activities including nonexercise activities, sleep information, and his perception of how he felt. After one month, Steve will return to the office for reevaluation and adjustments to his nutritional plan. Changes should reflect the level of progress made.

11.12 Conclusion

In this final chapter, we have taken all of the information learned in previous chapters and applied it to the case study of Steve, the powerlifter. We have examined the athletes presenting history including diet and workout plans. We have examined how Steve eats currently including trends and a 24-hour food recall. We have performed anthropometric tests to get a baseline for initiating the nutritional protocol. We worked with Steve to establish goals for him both in terms of his dietary desires as well as his goals for performance as a powerlifter. Next we determined the caloric needs for him to meet his goals. We calculated both his macro and micronutrient needs to support optimal performance. We developed a hydration strategy for him and a peri-workout nutritional plan. Finally we developed an initial supplementation plan targeted toward Steve's needs. From here, we send Steve out to follow the nutritional plan set out for him. We should plan to meet with Steve monthly to monitor progress and be prepared to make changes to the plan based on how he is performing.

References

1 McMurray RG, Soares J, Caspersen CJ, McCurdy T. Examining variations of resting metabolic rate of adults: a public health perspective. *Med. Sci. Sports Exerc.* 2014;46(7):1352–1358. doi:10.1249/MSS.0000000000000232
2 Joseph M, Gupta RD, Prema L, Inbakumari M, Thomas N. Are predictive equations for estimating resting energy expenditure accurate in Asian Indian male weightlifters?. *Indian J. Endocrinol. Metab.* 2017;21(4):515–519. doi:10.4103/ijem.IJEM_563_16
3 Jagim AR, Camic CL, Kisiolek J, et al. Accuracy of resting metabolic rate prediction equations in athletes. *J. Strength Cond. Res.* 2018;32(7):1875–1881. doi:10.1519/JSC.0000000000002111
4 Burke L, Deakin V. *Clinical Sports Nutrition.* 4th ed. McGraw-Hill Medical, 2010.

Index

24-hour food recall 99

a

A1C test 114
absorption rates, protein 154
acceptable macronutrient distribution range (AMDR), carbohydrates 43
acetyl-CoA 17–18
N-acetylcysteine (NAC) 164–165
active recovery techniques 147
activity multipliers 201–202
acute inflammation 140–141
adenosine diphosphate (ADP) 16
adenosine monophosphate (AMP) 16
adenosine triphosphate (ATP) 16–17, 16–22, 171
adequate intake (AI) 68
ADP *see* adenosine diphosphate
aerobic glycolysis 22
aging 27–37
  and athletic participation 2
  and endocrine system 30–34
  and motor neurons 29–30
  and oxygen delivery 34–35
  performance-based changes 28–29
  and physiology 1–2

AI *see* adequate intake
air displacement body fat analysis 109
alcohol consumption 32, 67
aldosterone 124
AMDR *see* acceptable macronutrient distribution range
amino acids 17, 50–51, 155–160
  beta-alanine 160
  branched chain 156–158, 174
  essential 157
  glutamine 159
  leucine 158
  ornithine 158–159
AMP *see* adenosine monophosphate
anabolic window 135
anabolism 18
anaerobic glycolysis 21–22
anthropometric testing 104–109
  air displacement body fat analysis 109
  bioelectric impedance 107–108
  body fat 107–109
  body measurements 105–109
  CT scans 109
  DEXA 108–109
  height 104–105
  hydrostatic weighing 108

Sports Nutrition for Masters Athletes, First Edition. Peter G. Nickless.
© 2025 John Wiley & Sons, Inc. Published 2025 by John Wiley & Sons, Inc.

Index

anthropometric testing (*cont'd*)
  MRI scans 109
  skinfold calipers 107
  weight 105
anti-diuretic hormone 31–32, 124
anti-inflammatory foods 144–146, 168–170
anti-inflammatory molecules 140
antioxidant-rich foods 145
antioxidant supplementation 164–165
arginine 159, 174
arsenic 67, 91
arthritis 178–179
ascorbic acid (vitamin C) 64–65, 77–78, 150–151
assessment
  anthropometric testing 104–109
  blood testing 114
  body fat 105–109
  client history 97–98
  dietary analysis 98–104
  dietary goals 193–195
  hydration 121–123, 10913
  performance metrics 195–196
  see also individual methods…
athletic population demographics 2
ATP *see* adenosine triphosphate

b

basal metabolic rate (BMR) 197–201
BCAAs *see* branched chain amino acids
beetroot 174
beta-alanine 160
beta-oxidation 17
biochemistry 13–26
  aerobic glycolysis 22
  anaerobic glycolysis 21–22
  beta-oxidation 17
  carbohydrates 40–43

energy production 15–16
energy systems 19–25
fats 56–60
gluconeogenesis 17
glycogenesis 18, 45
glycogenolysis 18–19, 45
glycolysis 17
homeostasis 14–15
inflammation 140–141
and intensity 22–24
ketogenesis 18
ketogenic diets 59–60
phosphagen system 20–21, 22
protein 50–52
in sports nutrition 16–19
tricarboxylic acid cycle 18
water 118
bioelectric impedance measurements 107–108
biological value, protein 50
biotin (vitamin B7) 64–65, 75–76
blood glucose testing 114
blood sugar
  glucagon 14–15, 18, 45
  glycemic index 45–47
  insulin 14–15, 18, 45, 131–132
blood tests 114
BMI *see* body mass index
BMR *see* basal metabolic rate
body fat measurements 105–109
  air displacement analysis 109
  anthropometric testing 109
  bioelectric impedance 107–108
  DEXA 108–109
  hydrostatic weighing 108
  MRI scans 109
  skinfold calipers 107
body mass index (BMI) 105
body measurements 105–106
body weight 105
  hydration testing 122

bones, supplementation support 177–179
boron 67, 91–92
Boswellia serrata 169–170
branched chain amino acids (BCAAs) 156–158, 174

c

caffeine 8, 172–173
calcium 66, 83–84
caloric requirements 9–10
  activity multipliers 201–202
  basal metabolic rate 197–201
  Cunningham formula 202
  determination 197–204
  rule-of-thumb methods 203
  thermic effect of activity 199
  thermic effect of food 199–200
calories 16
carbohydrate gels 161–162
carbohydrate loading 132–133
carbohydrate powders 161
carbohydrates 6, 40–49
  deficiencies 43–45
  disaccharides 41
  fiber 42–43
  glycemic index 45–47
  homeostasis 45
  and intensity 40
  intra-workout 133–134
  monosaccharides 41
  oligosaccharides 41–42
  polysaccharides 42
  post-exercise 135
  pre-exercise 130–133
  reactive hypoglycemia 131–132
  requirements 47–49
  structure 41–43
  supplementation 160–162
cartilage 178
casein 50–51, 154
catabolism 19
cellulose 42
chitosan 175
chloride 66, 82–83
cholecalciferol (vitamin D3) 79–80
cholesterol, and fiber 43
choline 93
chondroitin 178–179
chromium 66, 90, 174
chronic inflammation 141
citrulline 174
classification
  fats 56–57
  vitamins 64–66
client history 97–98
CoA *see* coenzyme A
cobalamin (vitamin B12) 64–65, 76–77
cobalt 67
coenzyme A (CoA) 73–74
complete blood count with differential 114
complex carbohydrates 41–43
computed tomography (CT), body fat analysis 109
copper 66, 88–89
cortisol 32–33, 143, 165–168
creatine monohydrate 170–171
creatine phosphate 20–21, 22
creation, nutritional plans 196–209
cryotherapy 147
CT *see* computed tomography
Cunningham formula 202
curcumin 169
cytokines 140

d

deficiencies, carbohydrates 43–45
dehydration 120–121
dehydroepiandrostendione (DHEA) 165–166

demographics   2
DEXA *see* dual-energy X-ray absorptiometry
dextrose   161
DHA *see* docosahexaenoic acid
DHEA *see* dehydroepiandrostendione
DIAAS *see* digestible indispensable amino acid score
dietary analysis   98–104
  24-hour food recall   99
  food diaries   99–100
  food frequency questionnaires   101–102
  indirect calorimetry   103
  instrument choice   102–103
dietary goals   8–9, 193–195
dietary reference intakes (DRI)   67–70
dietary water   119
digestibility, protein   50–51
digestible indispensable amino acid score (DIAAS)   50–51, 153–154
disaccharides   41
docosahexaenoic acid (DHA)   168–169
DRI *see* dietary reference intakes
dual-energy X-ray absorptiometry (DEXA)   108–109
Durnin and Womersley method   107
dynapenia   30

e

EAR *see* estimated average requirement
egg protein   154
eicosanoids   58
eicosapentaenoic acid (EPA)   168
electrolytes   66, 82–83
  hormonal regulation   124
  intra-workout   134
  laboratory tests   114
  sports drinks   125–126
  sweat analysis   109–113
  water balance   118
elements   7
  see also minerals; *specific elements...*
endocrine system
  and aging   30–34
  and stress   143
energy
  forms of   16
  production   15–16
energy systems   19–25
  aerobic glycolysis   22
  anaerobic glycolysis   21–22
  and intensity   22–24
  overview   20
  phosphagen system   20–21, 22
enrichment   70
environmental factors, inflammation   143
EPA *see* eicosapentaenoic acid
ephedrine   175
epinephrine   33
ergocalciferol (vitamin D2)   79–80
ergogenic supplementation   170–176
essential amino acids   157
essential fatty acids   58–59
essential trace minerals   66, 85–90
estimated average requirement (EAR)   68
estrogen   34
exercise, and inflammation   141–142

f

FAD *see* flavin adenine dinucleotide
fats   6, 55–60
  classifications   56–57
  essential   58–59
  hydrogenation   58
  and inflammation   58, 142
  ketogenic diets   59–60

omega-3/omega-6 58, 142, 145, 168–169
saturated 56
unsaturated 57
see also lipids
fat-soluble vitamins 65–66, 78–82
fatty acids 57–59
fiber 6, 42–43
fish oils 168–169
flavin adenine dinucleotide (FAD) 72
flavin mononucleotide (FMN) 72
fluids 119
fluoride 67, 91
FMN *see* flavin mononucleotide
FODMAP diet 42
folate 64–65, 76
food diaries 99–100
food frequency questionnaires 101–102
forms of energy 16
fortification 70
fructose 41, 134
functions of water 118–119

g

galactose 41
glucagon 14–15, 18, 45
gluconeogenesis 17
glucosamine 177–178
glucose 41
glutamine 159
glycemic index 45–47
glycemic load 46–47
glycerol 17
glycogen 14, 18, 42, 132–133
glycogenesis 18, 45
glycogenolysis 18–19, 45
glycolysis 17, 21–22
goals 8–9, 193–195
"golden hour" 135

growth-focused supplementation 151–160
growth hormone 31

h

Harris–Benedict equation 200
height measurement 104–105
herbs, anti-inflammatory 145
hierarchy of nutritional needs determination 9
high-sensitivity C-reactive reactive protein 114
histamine 140
homeostasis 14–15, 18, 118–119
hormones 6, 14–15, 18, 30–34, 165–168
  and aging 30–34
  androgens 34, 167–168
  carbohydrate metabolism 14–15, 18, 45, 131–132
  fatty acids 58
  stress 32–33, 143, 165–168
  supplementation 165–168
  thyroid 33–34, 114
  water balance 124
  see also specific hormones...
hydration 7, 10, 117–127
  assessment 109–113, 121–123
  during exercise 123–124
  functions of water 118–119
  hormonal regulation 124
  imbalance impacts 120–121
  inflammation management 146
  nonexercise sweat testing 113
  nutritional planning 206–207
  peri-workout 123–125
  pre-exercise 123
  sources of water 119
  sports drinks 125–126
  strategies 123–125, 206–207
  sweat analysis 109–110

hydration (cont'd)
   sweat rate test 110–112
   sweat sodium concentration 112–113
   and temperature regulation 118–119
   water loss 120
hydrogenation 58
hydrostatic weighing 108
hypoglycemia, reactive 131–132

i
indirect calorimetry 103
inflammation 139–148
   acute 140–141
   in athletes 141–143
   chronic 141
   dietary strategies 144–146
   environmental factors 143
   and exercise 141–142
   management 143–147
   and nutrition 58, 142
   omega-3/omega-6 58, 142, 145, 168–169
   physiology 140–141
   recovery techniques 146–147
   supplementation 146, 168–170, 178–179
insulin 14–15, 18, 45, 131–132
intensity
   and carbohydrates 40
   and energy systems 22–24
interleukins 140
intra-workout nutrition 123–124, 133–134
iodine 66, 87
iron 66, 85–86

j
joints, supplementation support 177–179

journaling, food diaries 99–100
junior athletes, definition 4

k
Katch–Mcardle equation 200–201
ketogenesis 18
ketogenic diets 59–60
ketone bodies 18
Krebs cycle 18, 22

l
laboratory testing 114
lactate 17
LDL *see* low-density lipoprotein
leucine 158
leukotrienes 140
linoleic acid 59
linolenic acid 59
lipid profiles 114
lipids 6
   classification 56–57
   see also fats
low-density lipoprotein (LDL) 44
luteinizing hormone 167

m
macronutrients 1, 6, 10, 39–61
   carbohydrates 6, 40–49, 130–135, 160–162
   fats 55–60, 142, 145, 168–169
   intra-workout 133–134
   ketogenic diets 59–60
   nutritional planning 204–206
   post-exercise 135
   pre-exercise 130–133
   protein 49–55, 135, 152–155
macrophages 140
magnesium 66, 84–85
magnetic resonance imaging (MRI), body fat analysis 109
major minerals 66, 83–85

maltodextrin 161
maltose 41
management, of inflammation 143–147
manganese 66, 89
margerine 58
massage 147
masters athletes
  definition 4
  specific needs 4–5
melatonin 32
menadione (vitamin K3) 80–81
menaquinone (vitamin K2) 80–81
metabolic water 119
metabolism 16–19
  activity multipliers 201–202
  basal rate 197–201
  carbohydrates 40–43
  fats 58–60
  ketogenic diets 59–60
  protein 50–52
  thermic effect of activity 199
  thermic effect of food 199–200
  see also biochemistry; physiology
methylsulfonylmethane (MSM) 179
microbiome supplementation 176–177
micronutrients 6–7, 10, 63–96
  dietary reference intakes 67–70
  electrolytes 66, 82–83
  essential trace minerals 66, 85–90
  fat-soluble vitamins 65–66, 78–82
  fortification and enrichment 70
  laboratory tests 114
  major minerals 66, 83–85
  multivitamins 162–163
  nonessential trace minerals 67, 91–93
  nutritional planning 206
  water-soluble vitamins 64–65, 70–78

  see also individual minerals, vitamins and electrolytes...
Mifflin-St. Jeor equation 200
milk protein 50–51, 154
minerals 7, 66, 83–93
  essential trace 66, 85–90
  laboratory tests 114
  major 66, 83–85
  nonessential trace 67, 91–93
  supplementation 162–163
  see also specific minerals...
molybdenum 66, 90
monosaccharides 41
monounsaturated fats 58
motor neurons 29–30
motor units 29–30
MRI *see* magnetic resonance imaging
MSM *see* methylsulfonylmethane
multivitamins 162–163
muscle-focused supplementation 151–160

n
NAC *see* N-acetylcysteine
negative feedback 14–15
nervous system
  and aging 29–30
  carbohydrates 44
neutrophils 140
niacin (vitamin B3) 64–65, 72–73
nickel 67, 92
nitric oxide 174
nitrogen balance 51–52
nonessential trace minerals 67, 91–93
nonexercise sweat testing 113
norepinephrine 33
nutritional needs
  assessment 97–116
  caloric requirements 9–10
  carbohydrates 40–49

nutritional needs (*cont'd*)
  diet, overview 8–10
  fats 55–60
  hierarchy of 9
  hydration 7, 117–127
  inflammation management 144–146
  macronutrients 6, 10, 39–61
  micronutrients 6–7, 10, 63–96
  overview 1–10, 5–10
  protein 49–55
  supplementation 7–8, 10
nutritional plans 191–209
  caloric needs determination 197–204
  creation 196–209
  dietary goals 193–195
  hydration 206–207
  macronutrients 204–206
  metrics 195–196
  micronutrients 206
  nutritional assessment 191–193
  peri-workout 207–208
  supplementation 208–209
nutrition assessment 97–116, 191–193
  anthropometric testing 104–109
  body fat 105–109
  case study 192–193
  client history 97–98
  dietary analysis 98–103
  hydration 109–113
  laboratory testing 114

o

oligosaccharides 41–42
omega-3/omega-6 58, 142, 145, 168–169
oranges 150–151
ornithine 158–159
osteoarthritis 178–179
oxidative stress 164–165

oxygen delivery
  and aging 34–35
  VO_2 max 35
oxytocin 14

p

pantothenic acid (vitamin B5) 64–65, 73–74
patch test 113
PDCAAS *see* protein digestibility corrected amino acid score
pea protein 154
performance
  and aging 28–29
  and carbohydrate deficiency 43–45
  and ketogenic diets 59–60
performance dietary plans 191–209
  caloric needs determination 197–204
  creation 196–209
  goals 193–195
  hydration 206–207
  macronutrients 204–206
  metrics 195–196
  micronutrients 206
  nutritional assessment 191–193
  nutritional plans 196–209
  nutrition assessment 192–193
  peri-workout 207–208
  supplementation 208–209
performance metrics 195–196
peri-workout nutrition 129–137
  carbohydrates 130–135
  electrolytes 134
  hydration 123–125
  intra-exercise 133–134
  plans 207–208
  post-exercise 134–135
  pre-workout 130–133
  protein 130, 135

phosphagen system 20–21, 22
phosphatidylserine 167–168
phospholipids 56
phosphorus 66, 84
phylloquinone (vitamin K1) 80–81
physiology 13–26
   aerobic glycolysis 22
   and aging 1–2, 28–29
   anaerobic glycolysis 21–22
   beta-oxidation 17
   carbohydrates 40–43
   energy production 15–16
   energy systems 19–25
   fats 56–60
   gluconeogenesis 17
   glycogenesis 18
   glycogenolysis 18–19
   glycolysis 17
   homeostasis 14–15
   and hydration 7, 10
   inflammation 140–141
   and intensity 22–24
   ketogenesis 18
   ketogenic diets 59–60
   phosphagen system 20–21, 22
   protein 50–52
   in sports nutrition 16–19
   tricarboxylic acid cycle 18
   water 118
plant-based protein 154–155
PLP *see* pyridoxal-5-phosphate
polysaccharides 42
polyunsaturated fats 58
positive feedback 14
post-exercise nutrition 124, 134–135
potassium 66, 83
prebiotic supplements 177
pre-exercise nutrition 123, 130–131, 176
primary sources, water 119
probiotics 177

pro-inflammatory foods 142
pro-inflammatory molecules 140
prostaglandins 140
protein 6, 49–55
   absorption rates 154
   digestibility 50–51
   and health 52–53
   nitrogen balance 51–52
   post-exercise 135
   pre-exercise 130
   quality assessment 50–51, 154–155
   requirements 53–55
   supplementation 152–155
protein digestibility corrected amino acid score (PDCAAS) 50–51
protein efficiency ratio 50
protein form 154–155
pyridoxal-5-phosphate (PLP) 74–75
pyridoxine (vitamin B6) 64–65, 74–75
pyruvate 17
pyruvic acid 17

q

quality assessment
   protein 50–51, 154–155
   supplementation 154–155, 179–180
quercetin 170

r

RDA *see* recommended daily allowance
reactive hypoglycemia 131–132
recommended daily allowance (RDA) 68
recovery techniques, inflammation management 146–147
repair-focused supplementation 151–160

requirements
  carbohydrates 48
  micronutrients 67–70
  protein 53–55
retinol (vitamin A) 65
riboflavin (vitamin B2) 64–65, 72
rule-of-thumb methods, caloric requirements 203

s

saponins 167
sarcopenia 30
saturated fats 57–58
selenium 66, 88
senior athletes, definition 4
serum albumin 114
shellfish allergies 178
shivering 110, 119
silicon 67, 92–93
simple amino acid score 50
simple carbohydrates 41
skinfold caliper measurements 107
sleep 146
sodium 66, 82
  hormonal regulation 124
  sweat concentration 112–113
sodium bicarbonate 171–172
somatotrophin 31
sources of water 119
soy protein 50–51
spices, anti-inflammatory 145, 169
sports drinks 125–126
sports nutrition
  biochemical reactions 16–19
  concepts 3
  reasons for study 3–4
starch 42
sterols 56
stress 143
sucrose 41
supercompensation 132–133

supplementation 7–8, 10, 149–190
  amino acids 155–160
  bone and joint support 177–179
  carbohydrate powders and gels 160–162
  ergogenic 170–176
  hormonal balance 165–168
  inflammation management 146, 168–170, 178–179
  microbiome 176–177
  nutritional plans 208–209
  osteoarthritis 178–179
  overview 149–150
  oxidative stress 164–165
  pre-workout 176
  protein 152–155
  quality 154–155, 179–180
  repair and growth 151–160
  vitamins and minerals 162–163
  vs whole foods 150–151
sweat analysis 109–110
sweating 118–119
sweat rate test 110–112
sweat sodium concentration 112–113

t

T3/T4 hormones 33–34
tart cherry juice 170
TCA cycle *see* tricarboxylic acid cycle
TCR *see* total caloric requirements
TEA *see* thermic effect of activity
TEF *see* thermic effect of food
temperature homeostasis 118–119
testosterone 34, 167–168
tetrahydrofolate (THF) 76
thermic effect of activity (TEA) 199
thermic effect of food (TEF) 199–200
thermoregulation 118–119
THF *see* tetrahydrofolate

thiamin (vitamin B1)   64–65, 71
thyroid hormones   33–34
thyroid panels   114
tolerable upper intake levels
   (ULs)   69
total caloric requirements
   (TCR)   197
trace minerals   66–67
trans fats   58, 142
Tribulus terrestris   167
tricarboxylic acid cycle (TCA cycle)
   18, 22
triglycerides   56–57
tumor necrosis factor-alpha   140
turmeric   169
type 2 diabetes   124–125

u

ULs *see* tolerable upper intake levels
unsaturated fats   58
urine testing, hydration   122–123

v

vanadium   67, 93
vasodilation, and inflammation   140
vasopressin   31–32, 124
vitamin A (retinol)   65, 78–79
vitamin B1 (thiamin)   64–65, 71
vitamin B2 (riboflavin)   64–65, 72
vitamin B3 (niacin)   64–65, 72–73
vitamin B5 (pantothenic acid)
   64–65, 73–74
vitamin B6 (pyridoxine)   64–65,
   74–75
vitamin B7 (biotin)   64–65, 75–76
vitamin B12 (cobalamin)   64–65,
   76–77

vitamin C (ascorbic acid)   64–65,
   77–78, 150–151
vitamin D   65, 79–80, 151
vitamin E   65, 81–82
vitamin H   64–65, 75–76
vitamin K   65, 80–81
vitamins   7
   fat-soluble   65–66, 78–82
   laboratory tests   114
   overview   63–64
   supplementation   162–163
   water-soluble   64–65, 70–78
VO_2 max   35

w

waist-to-hip measurement   106
warfarin   178
water
   in the body   118
   functions of   118–119
   hormonal regulation   124
   loss   120
   sources of   119
water-soluble vitamins   64–65, 70–78
weight loss, supplementation
   170–176
weight measurement   105
whey protein   50–51, 154–155, 158
whole-body wash-down
   technique   112–113

x

X-rays, body fat measurements
   108–109

z

zinc   66, 86–87